Pediatric Immunology and Allergy

Editor

ELIZABETH SECORD

PEDIATRIC CLINICS
OF NORTH AMERICA

www.pediatric.theclinics.com

Consulting Editor
BONITA F. STANTON

October 2019 • Volume 66 • Number 5

ELSEVIER

1600 John F. Kennedy Boulevard • Suite 1800 • Philadelphia, Pennsylvania, 19103-2899

http://www.theclinics.com

THE PEDIATRIC CLINICS OF NORTH AMERICA Volume 66, Number 5
October 2019 ISSN 0031-3955, ISBN-13: 978-0-323-67892-6

Editor: Kerry Holland
Developmental Editor: Casey Potter

The Pediatric Clinics of North America (ISSN 0031-3955) is published bimonthly by Elsevier Inc., 360 Park Avenue South, New York, NY 10010-1710. Months of issue are February, April, June, August, October, and December. Periodicals postage paid at New York, NY and additional mailing offices. Subscription prices are $229.00 per year (US individuals), $653.00 per year (US institutions), $315.00 per year (Canadian individuals), $868.00 per year (Canadian institutions), $345.00 per year (international individuals), $868.00 per year (international institutions), $100.00 per year (US students and residents), and $165.00 per year (international and Canadian residents and students). To receive students/resident rare, orders must be accompanied by name of affiliated institution, date of term, and the signature of program/residency coordinator on institution letterhead. Orders will be billed at individual rate until proof of status is received. Foreign air speed delivery is included in all *Clinics* subscription prices. All prices are subject to change without notice. **POSTMASTER:** Send address changes to *The Pediatric Clinics of North America*, Elsevier Health Sciences Division, Subscription Customer Service, 3251 Riverport Lane, Maryland Heights, MO 63043. **Customer Service: 1-800-654-2452 (US and Canada). From outside of the US and Canada: 1-314-447-8871. Fax: 1-314-447-8029. For print support, E-mail: JournalsCustomerService-usa@elsevier.com. For online support, E-mail: JournalsOnlineSupport-usa@elsevier.com.**

Reprints. For copies of 100 or more, of articles in this publication, please contact the Commercial Reprints Department, Elsevier Inc., 360 Park Avenue South, New York, NY 10010-1710. Tel.: 212-633-3874; Fax: 212-633-3820; E-mail: reprints@elsevier.com.

The Pediatric Clinics of North America is also published in Spanish by McGraw-Hill Inter-americana Editores S.A., Mexico City, Mexico; in Portuguese by Riechmann and Affonso Editores, Rua Comandante Coelho 1085, CEP 21250, Rio de Janeiro, Brazil; and in Greek by Althayia SA, Athens, Greece.

The Pediatric Clinics of North America is covered in *MEDLINE/PubMed (Index Medicus), Excerpta Medica, Current Contents, Current Contents/Clinical Medicine, Science Citation Index, ASCA, ISI/BIOMED,* and *BIOSIS.*

PROGRAM OBJECTIVE

The goal of the *Pediatric Clinics of North America* is to keep practicing physicians and residents up to date with current clinical practice in pediatrics by providing timely articles reviewing the state-of-the-art in patient care.

TARGET AUDIENCE

All practicing pediatricians, physicians and healthcare professionals who provide patient care to pediatric patients.

LEARNING OBJECTIVES

Upon completion of this activity, participants will be able to:
1. Review new targeted therapies for the treatment of asthma.
2. Discuss current and emerging food allergy prevention strategies, diagnostic tools, and potential treatments.
3. Recognize common pediatric drug allergies and methods for diagnosis.

ACCREDITATIONS
Physician Credit

The Elsevier Office of Continuing Medical Education (EOCME) is accredited by the Accreditation Council for Continuing Medical Education (ACCME) to provide continuing medical education for physicians.

The EOCME designates this journal-based activity for a maximum of 12 *AMA PRA Category 1 Credit*(s)™. Physicians should claim only the credit commensurate with the extent of their participation in the activity.

All other healthcare professionals requesting continuing education credit for this this journal-based activity will be issued a certificate of participation.

ABP Maintenance of Certification Credit

Successful completion of this CME activity, which includes participation in the activity and individual assessment of and feedback to the learner, enables the learner to earn up to 12 MOC points in the American Board of Pediatrics' (ABP). Maintenance of Certification (MOC) program. It is the CME activity provider's responsibility to submit learner completion information to ACCME for the purpose of granting ABP MOC credit.

DISCLOSURE OF CONFLICTS OF INTEREST

The EOCME assesses conflict of interest with its instructors, faculty, planners, and other individuals who are in a position to control the content of CME activities. All relevant conflicts of interest that are identified are thoroughly vetted by EOCME for fair balance, scientific objectivity, and patient care recommendations. EOCME is committed to providing its learners with CME activities that promote improvements or quality in healthcare and not a specific proprietary business or a commercial interest.

The planning committee, staff, authors and editors listed below have identified no financial relationships or relationships to products or devices they or their spouse/life partner have with commercial interest related to the content of this CME activity:
Matthew Adams, MD; Heather Axelrod, DO; Marwa El-Bohy, MD; Kerry Holland; Jenny Huang, MD; Bani Preet Kaur, MD; Alison Kemp; David A. Khan, MD; Weyman Lam, MD; Heather K. Lehman, MD; Shazia Lutfeali, MD; Rajkumar Mayakrishnan; Tayaba Miah, MD; Jenny Maribel Montejo, MD; Roxanne Carbonell Oriel, MD; Milind Pansare, MD; Pavadee Poowuttikul, MD; Shweta Saini, MD; Charles Frank Schuler IV, MD; Elizabeth Secord, MD; Divya Seth, MD; Bonita F. Stanton, MD; Mohammed Taki, MD; Julie Wang, MD

UNAPPROVED/OFF-LABEL USE DISCLOSURE

The EOCME requires CME faculty to disclose to the participants:
1. When products or procedures being discussed are off-label, unlabelled, experimental, and/or investigational (not US Food and Drug Administration [FDA] approved); and
2. Any limitations on the information presented, such as data that are preliminary or that represent ongoing research, interim analyses, and/or unsupported opinions. Faculty may discuss information about pharmaceutical agents that is outside of FDA-approved labelling. This information is intended solely for CME and is not intended to promote off-label use of these medications. If you have any questions, contact the medical affairs department of the manufacturer for the most recent prescribing information.

TO ENROLL

To enroll in the *Pediatric Clinics of North America* Continuing Medical Education program, call customer service at 1-800-654-2452 or sign up online at http://www.theclinics.com/home/cme. The CME program is available to subscribers for an additional annual fee of USD 301.60.

METHOD OF PARTICIPATION

In order to claim credit, participants must complete the following:

1. Complete enrolment as indicated above.
2. Read the activity.
3. Complete the CME Test and Evaluation. Participants must achieve a score of 70% on the test. All CME Tests and Evaluations must be completed online.

In order to claim MOC points, participants must complete the following:

1. Complete steps listed above for claiming CME credit
2. Provide your specialty board ID#, birth date (MM/DD), and attestation.
3. Online MOC submission is only available for the American Board of Pediatrics' (ABP) Maintenance of Certification (MOC) program

CME INQUIRIES/SPECIAL NEEDS

For all CME inquiries or special needs, please contact elsevierCME@elsevier.com

Contributors

CONSULTING EDITOR

BONITA F. STANTON, MD
Founding Dean, Hackensack Meridian School of Medicine at Seton Hall University, President, Academic Enterprise, Hackensack Meridian Health Robert C. and Laura C. Garrett Endowed Chair for the School of Medicine, Professor of Pediatrics, Nutley, New Jersey

EDITOR

ELIZABETH SECORD, MD
Professor of Pediatrics, Division of Allergy and Immunology, Department of Pediatrics, Children's Hospital of Michigan, Wayne State University, Detroit, Michigan

AUTHORS

MATTHEW ADAMS, MD
Division of Pediatric Rheumatology, Department of Pediatrics, Children's Hospital of Michigan, Wayne State University, Detroit, Michigan

HEATHER AXELROD, MD
Department of Pediatrics (PGY3), Children's Hospital of Michigan, Detroit, Michigan

MARWA EL-BOHY, MD
Division of Allergy and Immunology, Department of Pediatrics, Children's Hospital of Michigan, Wayne State University, Detroit, Michigan

JENNY HUANG, MD
Fellow, Department of Allergy Immunology, Children's Hospital of Michigan, Wayne State University, Detroit, Michigan

BANI PREET KAUR, MD
Detroit Medical Center, Children's Hospital of Michigan, Detroit, Michigan

DAVID A. KHAN, MD
Department of Internal Medicine, Division of Allergy and Immunology, The University of Texas Southwestern Medical Center, Dallas, Texas

WEYMAN LAM, MD
Division of Allergy, Immunology, and Rheumatology, Department of Pediatrics, Jacobs School of Medicine and Biomedical Sciences, University at Buffalo, Buffalo, New York

HEATHER K. LEHMAN, MD
Division of Allergy, Immunology, and Rheumatology, Department of Pediatrics, Jacobs School of Medicine and Biomedical Sciences, University at Buffalo, Buffalo, New York

SHAZIA LUTFEALI, MD
Department of Internal Medicine, Division of Allergy and Immunology, The University of Texas Southwestern Medical Center, Dallas, Texas

TAYABA MIAH, MD
Resident, Department of Pediatrics, Children's Hospital of Michigan, Detroit, Michigan

JENNY MARIBEL MONTEJO, MD
Clinical Assistant Professor, Division of Allergy and Clinical Immunology, University of Michigan, Domino's Farms, Ann Arbor, Michigan

ROXANNE CARBONELL ORIEL, MD
Assistant Professor, Department of Pediatrics, Division of Allergy and Immunology, Icahn School of Medicine at Mount Sinai, New York, New York

MILIND PANSARE, MD
Division of Allergy and Immunology, Department of Pediatrics, Children's Hospital of Michigan, Pediatric Specialty Center, Assistant Professor, Clinician Educator, Wayne State University, Detroit, Michigan

PAVADEE POOWUTTIKUL, MD
Associate Professor of Pediatrics, Division of Allergy and Immunology, Allergy/Immunology Fellowship Training Program Director, Children's Hospital of Michigan, Wayne State University School of Medicine, Detroit, Michigan

SHWETA SAINI, MD
Division of Hospital Medicine, Fellow-in-Training, Division of Allergy and Immunology, Department of Pediatrics, Children's Hospital of Michigan, Wayne State University School of Medicine, Detroit, Michigan

CHARLES FRANK SCHULER IV, MD
Fellow, Division of Allergy and Clinical Immunology, University of Michigan, Domino's Farms, Ann Arbor, Michigan

ELIZABETH SECORD, MD
Professor of Pediatrics, Division of Allergy and Immunology, Department of Pediatrics, Children's Hospital of Michigan, Wayne State University, Detroit, Michigan

DIVYA SETH, MD
Assistant Professor, Clinical Educator, Division of Allergy/Immunology, Department of Pediatrics, Children's Hospital of Michigan, Wayne State University School of Medicine, Detroit, Michigan

MOHAMMED TAKI, MD
Resident, Department of Pediatrics, Children's Hospital of Michigan, Detroit, Michigan

JULIE WANG, MD
Professor, Department of Pediatrics, Division of Allergy and Immunology, Icahn School of Medicine at Mount Sinai, New York, New York

Contents

The most common primary immune deficiencies are those of the humoral immune system, and most of these present in childhood. The severity of these disorders ranges from transient deficiencies to deficiencies that are associated with a complete loss of ability to make adequate or functional antibodies, and have infectious as well as noninfectious complications. This article reviews, in a case-based discussion, the most common of the humoral immune deficiencies; their presentations, diagnoses, treatments; and, when known, the genetic defects.

The innate immune response system forms an important line of defense by deploying a limited number of receptors specific for conserved microbial components. This deployment generates a rapid inflammatory response, while activating the adaptive immune system. Improvements in our understanding of the innate immune system have allowed us to explore various therapeutic strategies via modulation of the immune response.

The T-cell receptor excision circle (TREC) assay is an effective screening tool for severe combined immunodeficiency (SCID). The TREC assay was designed to detect typical SCID and leaky SCID, but any condition causing low naïve T-cell counts will also be detected. Newborn screening for SCID using the TREC assay has proven itself to be highly sensitive and cost-efficient. This review covers the history of SCID newborn screening, elaborates on the SCID subtypes and TREC assay limitations, and discusses diagnostic and management considerations for infants with a positive screen.

Asthma is a complex, heterogeneous chronic airway disease with high prevalence of uncontrolled disease. New therapies, including biologics, are now available to treat T2 high asthma. Treatment of T2 low asthma remains a challenge. Asthma guidelines need be to updated to incorporate new therapeutics.

rhinorrhea, nasal obstruction, and nasal itching. When the eyes are involved, the term allergic rhinoconjunctivitis is used. Triggers may include airborne pollens, molds, dust mites, and animals. Skin or blood allergy testing can be a useful diagnostic modality that may guide therapy. Immunotherapy can prevent the development of further allergic sensitizations as well as subsequent asthma.

Anaphylaxis is an acute, potentially life-threatening systemic hypersensitivity reaction. Classically, anaphylaxis is an immunoglobulin (Ig) E–mediated reaction; however, IgG or immune complex complement-related immunologic reactions that lead to degranulation of mast cells can also cause anaphylaxis. Food allergy is the most common cause of anaphylaxis, followed by drugs. Patients with anaphylaxis commonly present with symptoms involving skin or mucous membranes, followed by respiratory and gastrointestinal symptoms. Epinephrine is the drug of choice for treating anaphylaxis. Patients and caregivers should be educated on the use of epinephrine autoinjectors with periodic review of symptoms and emergency action plan for anaphylaxis.

Biologics are protein-based pharmaceuticals derived from living organisms or their proteins. We discuss the mechanism of action for currently approved biologics and a give summary of the studies on immune suppression from biologics. Most of these studies have been conducted with rheumatology patients, and many in adults. Their relevance for children is explored and existing gaps in data for children are highlighted.

Atopic dermatitis is a complex, chronic inflammatory skin disorder with significant morbidity. It is often a frustrating condition for both children and parents due to chronic and relapsing course. There is now an increasing understanding of the disease pathogenesis resulting in discovery of much wanted newer therapeutics and targeted therapies after a long time. Whether these interventions will result in sustained benefits or long term cure remains to be seen.

Adverse drug reactions are frequently reported in pediatric patients. In this review article, the authors discuss pediatric drug allergies with emphasis on the most common culprits, beta-lactam antibiotics and non-steroidal anti-inflammatory drugs. The authors also discuss reactions to non-beta-lactam antibiotics and chemotherapeutics. Skin testing has not yet been validated for many drugs, although notable exceptions include penicillin and carboplatin. The gold standard for diagnosis in most cases remains drug challenge, and the need for penicillin skin testing prior to oral provocation challenge has been questioned in recent studies. Successful desensitizations have also been reported with several drugs.

PEDIATRIC CLINICS OF NORTH AMERICA

SERIES OF RELATED INTEREST

Clinics in Perinatology
https://www.perinatology.theclinics.com/
Advances in Pediatrics
https://www.advancesinpediatrics.com/

THE CLINICS ARE AVAILABLE ONLINE!
Access your subscription at:
www.theclinics.com

Foreword

The Ever-Expanding Base of New Knowledge

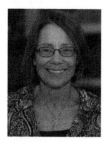

Bonita F. Stanton, MD
Consulting Editor

This issue of *Pediatric Clinics of North America* clearly illustrates why medical schools in the twenty-first century are actively seeking new ways to teach medicine. As noted by Dr Secord in her preface, there have been remarkable changes in our understanding of many of the basic premises of allergy and immunology, with significant advances in treatment accompanying this new understanding. This proliferation of new knowledge is certainly not limited to immunology and allergy; rather, it is being seen across the field of medicine. It is estimated that the doubling time of medical knowledge in 1950 was 50 years, decreasing to 3.5 years in 2010. It is predicted that by the year 2020, it will be just 73 days. Our current medical students will have experienced approximately 4 doublings of knowledge while in medical school. It is no longer possible—or desirable—to rely simply on memory; students must learn how to continually learn, as they will need to do during the remainder of their medical careers. Advances in the field of allergy and immunology clearly illustrate the rapidity of our changing understanding of the pathogenesis of disease, and correspondingly, our treatment and prevention.[1]

In recent years we have learned that over half of premature deaths are due to non-biologic factors, even if ultimately these factors act through biologic paths.[2] Certainly, many of the causes of illness, including death, resulting from the allergic and immunologic diseases described herein by Dr Secord and her colleagues result from a combination of external and internal causes, which are both biologic and nonbiologic. This need to understand the intersection of biologic stress and disorders with environmental challenges is clearly described in these articles.

The message across these articles signals the need for a broadening of the informational platform that today's pediatricians and other pediatric health care providers must master to enable them to adequately engage in the lifelong learning that must characterize their medical careers. But regardless of his or her career stage, any child

Pediatr Clin N Am 66 (2019) xiii–xiv
https://doi.org/10.1016/j.pcl.2019.07.002
0031-3955/19/© 2019 Published by Elsevier Inc.

health provider reading these articles will come away with a good of understanding of contemporary pediatric allergic and immunologic practice.

Bonita F. Stanton, MD
Hackensack Meridian School of Medicine
at Seton Hall University
Academic Enterprise
340 Kingsland Street, Building 123
Nutley, NJ 07110, USA

E-mail address:
bonita.stanton@shu.edu

REFERENCES

1. Densen P. Challenges and opportunities facing medical education. Trans Am Clin Climatol Assoc 2011;122:48–58.
2. Schroeder SA. We can do better—improving the health of the American people. N Engl J Med 2007;357:1221–8.

Preface

Pediatric Immunology and Allergy

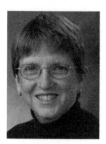

Elizabeth Secord, MD
Editor

This issue of *Pediatric Clinics of North America* focuses on some of the radical changes that have occurred in our field over the past few years and addresses some of the issues we still need to tackle. Food allergy prevention now involves early tolerance induction rather than avoidance of highly allergenic foods. Eosinophilic gut disease has its own set of practice parameters that differ for children and adults, and treatments are rapidly evolving for this disorder. Children with food allergies are now routinely challenged with the offending food, and in some cases, desensitized.

Severe combined immune deficiencies are now on the newborn screening panel in all 50 states. The current treatment of choice for confirmed severe combined immunodeficiency (SCID) is bone marrow or stem cell transplant. By the next time allergy and immunology is due for a *Pediatric Clinics of North America* rotation, many children with SCID will, if the current trajectory continues, be treated by gene therapy, which has already been piloted for some types of SCID.

Biologics are increasingly utilized to intervene in and modify immune dysregulation. Although these agents lead to some secondary immune deficiency, it appears to be less than originally feared. Rheumatologic conditions are probably the broadest set of disorders treated with biologics, but there is no specialty untouched by these rapidly evolving drugs, including asthma, atopic dermatitis, and chronic urticaria.

Asthma is no longer 1 disease, and targeted treatment is now becoming a reality. The biggest obstacles for the most severe asthmatics, however, remain social and environmental issues. Addressing these issues that continue to increase morbidity and mortality for our most vulnerable inner-city asthmatics is the greatest challenge

Pediatr Clin N Am 66 (2019) xv–xvi
https://doi.org/10.1016/j.pcl.2019.07.001
0031-3955/19/© 2019 Published by Elsevier Inc.

facing us today. I hope that by the time the next set of reviews for our specialty come around that we have made strides toward addressing these issues as well.

Elizabeth Secord, MD
Department of Pediatrics
Children's Hospital of Michigan
Wayne State University
3950 Beaubien Boulevard
Detroit, MI 48202, USA

E-mail address:
esecord@med.wayne.edu

Humoral Immune Deficiencies of Childhood

Marwa El-Bohy, MD, Pavadee Poowuttikul, MD, Elizabeth Secord, MD*

KEYWORDS

- Humoral immune deficiency • Immunoglobulin deficiency • B cell deficiency
- Antibody deficiency

KEY POINTS

- Humoral immune deficiencies are the most common immune deficiencies.
- Humoral immune deficiencies most commonly manifest in early childhood.
- Humoral immune deficiencies range from transient deficiencies to life-threatening deficiencies that require lifetime treatment.
- Humoral immune deficiencies diagnosis can be delayed if a high index of suspicion is not maintained or if the noninfectious manifestations are not appreciated.

CASE 1

Eleanor is 9 months old and is brought to her pediatrician because she has a cough and runny nose. Her mother is concerned that Eleanor is sick too often. She has had 3 colds, and 2 ear infections that were both treated with antibiotics. There is no family history of primary immune deficiency and she was born full term. Newborn T-cell receptor excision circle (TREC) screening for severe combined immune deficiencies was normal, and she does not have failure to thrive. Examination is normal except for rhinorrhea and a dry cough. There is no rash, no hepatomegaly, lungs are clear, and tonsillar tissue is present. Initial immune work-up reveals a negative human immunodeficiency virus (HIV) antibody test, an immunoglobulin (Ig) A level less than 7 mg/dL, an IgG of 147 mg/dL (lower limit of normal for age is 217 mg/dL), and IgM is in the normal range.

During the last trimester of pregnancy, fetuses are recipients of passive IgG from their mothers, and this cross-placental transfer protects infants for the first months of life.[1] Preterm infants have lower levels of IgG than full-term infants because they miss part or all of the placental transfer in the third trimester. Infants begin to make

Conflict of Interest: The authors declare no relevant conflict of interest.
Division of Allergy and Immunology, Department of Pediatrics, Children's Hospital of Michigan, Wayne State University, 3950 Beaubien Boulevard, Detroit, MI 48201, USA
* Corresponding author.
E-mail address: esecord@med.wayne.edu

their own IgG at birth, and the levels increase over the first few years of life. Maternal-transferred IgG level decreases to reach a nadir around 4 to 6 months of age.[1–5] Infants who do not begin to make their own immunoglobulin and their own specific antibody responses often start to show signs of increased infection and the sequelae of increased infection, such as failure to thrive, around 6 to 9 months of age.[3]

IgA deficiency is physiologic in infants.[5] IgA is present on mucosal surfaces and in secretions to protect the body from inhaled and ingested pathogens. Secretions such as saliva and breast milk contain high levels of IgA, and breastmilk provides passive transfer for the infant's gut.[2,3,5] However, IgA does not cross the placenta, and infants do not begin to make detectable levels of serum IgA until they are about 2 years of age.[5]

IgM is the first immunoglobulin expressed during B-cell development, and the first to be produced in the serum.[2] IgM antibodies are pentamers involved in the primary immune response, and as such are used as marker of acute infection. IgM production begins early, at about 24 weeks' gestation.[2–4]

The clinician realizes that the absent IgA is expected, is are worried about the low IgG level because this is a full-term infant. The clinician orders lymphocyte subsets and recall antibodies to pneumococci, tetanus, and diphtheria to further evaluate.

B lymphocytes possesses the unique quality of single-antigen specificity, contributing to the individualized, specific, and targeted response to each antigen encountered.[2–4] This large repertoire of antigen-specific receptors is mediated by recombination of DNA segments during maturation of lymphocytes. This process involves an almost random mixing of 3 regions of gene segments (variable, diversity, and joining regions). The rearrangement of DNA segments creates a great deal of diversity, and a process that introduces allowable error into the joining introduces further diversity. The entire process ensures recognition of a huge number of microbes.[2–4]

The immature B cell is identified by the IgM antibody on the surface. The next identifiable immunoglobulin present on maturing B cells is membrane-bound IgD. Immature B cells leaving the bone marrow are IgM⁺IgD⁺ and are then destined for secondary lymphoid organs to complete their maturation.[2–4] Once the immature B cell exits the bone marrow, the final stage of development occurs when it interacts with an antigen.[2] Although there are some T cell–independent antigens that can elicit an antibody response, almost all antibody responses require T-cell participation.[3,4]

B cells require 2 main signals for activation, the first of which is cross-linking of the immunoglobulin receptor, which occurs after antigens complex with IgM or IgG on the cell surface.[2] Once this cross-linking occurs, intracellular pathways are activated and prime the cell for interaction with T cells. This interaction occurs at the interface of primary follicles of lymphoid tissue (where the B cells reside) and the paracortical areas (where the T cells reside). Involvement of many costimulator molecules, such as cluster of differentiation (CD) 40, B7-1 (CD80), and B7-2 (CD86), come together to form the immunologic synapse, similar to that of the T cell receptor (TCR).[2] Once activated, most B cells enter the germinal center where class switching takes place to produce IgA, IgD, and IgE. This process occurs under cytokine control by a process of gene rearrangements to create genes that encode each immunoglobulin isotype. For example, IL-4 and IL-13 promote switching to IgE and IL-10 and transforming growth factor beta promote switching to IgA.[2,3,6,7]

The primary response to an antigen leads to production of predominantly IgM and is a slow response.[2] The secondary response is promoted by memory B and T cells, which allows for development of higher-affinity antibodies, including IgA, IgG, and IgE, in the later phase of the immune response.[2–4]

Lymphocyte enumeration results reveal normal numbers and percentages of CD3+ T cells, CD4+ T cells, CD8+ T cells, CD3-CD56+CD16+natural killer (NK) cells, and CD19+ B cells. Antibodies to pneumococci, tetanus, and diphtheria are adequate. The evidence now supports a diagnosis of transient hypogammaglobulinemia of infancy.

Transient hypogammaglobulinemia of infancy is often considered a normal variant, but sometimes this diagnosis confounds a work-up for immune deficiency in a child who has frequent upper respiratory infections and otitis media. Is this disorder causative or coincidental? It is not clear, but there is no role for replacement IgG in these children who do make functional antibody, as shown by adequate antibody responses to various antigens, and who usually recover and have normal or near-normal levels of IgG by 18 months to 3 years of age. It is common to see some of these children with slightly low IgG levels with normal antibody production for 5 to 6 years.[8] Following carefully and obtaining serial immunoglobulin and antibody levels is prudent to ensure that IgG level is increasing and to ensure that the antibody seen on the laboratory tests is truly the child's and not placental transfer. With more sensitive antibody tests, placental transfer may be detected beyond the 6-month mark, at which point most textbooks indicate that it should be gone. HIV is a good example. Transplacental transfer of HIV antibody is often detected as late as 18 months of age.[9]

CASE 2

Franklin is 4 years old and is brought to the pediatrician because he has a fever, a persistent cough, and an earache. His mother is concerned that he is sick too often. He has had pneumonia 3 times but has not been hospitalized. He is described as "always" having a cold with thick nasal secretions, and he has at least 5 ear infections a year. He has no family history of immune deficiency, and his mother reports no miscarriages before or after the birth of this child. Franklin was born full term. Newborn TREC screening for severe combined immune deficiencies was normal near birth, but he is below the fifth percentile for weight and height.[10] His poor weight gain has always been attributed to his poor appetite from frequent antibiotic use. Examination reveals a small boy with increased respiratory rate at 24 breaths/min and fever of 40°C. He has crackles on the right posterior lung field, no rash, and no hepatomegaly. Both tympanic membranes are scarred and pus is present in the left ear canal, and the right tympanic membrane is bulging and dull. No tonsillar tissue is appreciated.

His chest radiograph reveals a right middle lobe consolidation. He is admitted for intravenous (IV) antibiotic and responds rapidly. He is afebrile within 24 hours, but the inpatient team requests an immunologic work-up.

Initial immune work-up reveals a negative HIV antibody test, an IgA level less than 7 mg/dL, and undetectable IgG and IgM. Recall antibodies are absent to tetanus, diphtheria, and pneumococcus. His lymphocyte enumeration shows normal percentage and absolute count for all T-cell markers and NK cell markers, but CD19 B cells are absent. X-linked agammaglobulinemia (Bruton tyrosine kinase [BTK] deficiency) is suspected and genetic testing is ordered.

Agammaglobulinemia is most often X-linked and is caused by a genetic mutation in the BTK that leads to a block in the B-cell development from pre-B to immature B cell.[3,8] Other forms of agammaglobulinemia that are autosomal recessive have been identified, including some mutations in the heavy chain of the IgM molecule, which also stops B-cell maturation at the pre-B cell stage. Defects in the pre-B cell receptor, or mutations in the B cell linker protein, which is associated with the BTK protein, can also lead to autosomal recessive forms of agammaglobulinemia.[11–14] The presentation of the disease with increased infection and failure to thrive is similar to those of X-linked agammaglobulinemia. Although genetic testing for most of these autosomal recessive variants has recently become available commercially, it is also prudent to realize that just because a defect has not been identified does not mean that a disorder is not genetic. New genetic variants of primary immune deficiencies are being discovered at an increased frequency now because of accessibility of genetic testing.

Because antibiotics are used more frequently and earlier in the course of infection than was once true, the presentation of agammaglobulinemia can be delayed, and although classically patients with agammaglobulinemia lack tonsils, it is often a missed cue on physical examination. Current newborn screening does not detect B-cell deficiencies without associated T-cell defects. An investigational assay to detect B-cell defects at birth (kappa-deleting excision circles) may be added to newborn screening.[15]

The treatment of agammaglobulinemia includes replacement IgG, either IV (introduced in the 1980s to replace intramuscular product introduced in the 1950s) or subcutaneous (SC), which was introduced into general use in the 1990s.[16] The product, either IV or SC, comprises pooled IgG from multiple persons and is processed by cold ethanol fractionation combined with questionnaires and screening of donors to avoid most infectious agents.[16] A frequent clinical error in patients on IgG replacement is forgetting that antibody tests do not identify what the patient has been exposed to, and identify only what the plasma donors make. Laboratory tests that rely on antibodies are not useful for diagnosing infection in patients with agammaglobulinemia or in other patients who do not make their own antibodies.

IgA and IgM cannot be replaced because they are not as stable as IgG, and products for replacement of these immunoglobulin classes do not exist at this time, which leaves the patients more vulnerable to mucosal infection, especially gut and sinus infections. Patients with agammaglobulinemia should also be monitored for infection and treated with antibiotics promptly when appropriate. Persons with agammaglobulinemia have some increased risk of autoimmune disease and malignancy, although not so much as persons with common variable immune deficiency, which carries a higher degree of immune dysregulation.[17]

Franklin's genetic testing reveals the suspected defect in the BTK gene and he is continued on replacement Ig. The family decides to switch to home subcutaneous product. His IgG level is monitored at every 2 to 3 month intervals to assure adequate levels are maintained in this growing child. He is monitored at least twice yearly for adequate growth and to assess for any autoimmune complications.

CASE 3

Jimmy is 6 years old and presents for his yearly visit. His mother is concerned that he has frequent ear infections (4–5 yearly), and "always has a cold." He has received very few of his routine immunizations because he has always been sick at the time they should have been administered. On examination he does not have failure to thrive, does have tonsils, and has no hepatomegaly. His tympanic membranes are without scars, but they are dull. He has postnasal drip and nasal congestion. Immunoglobulins are obtained and recall antigens for tetanus, diphtheria, and pneumococci. The IgG and IgM levels are within normal limits, but IgA is less than 7 mg/dL and although his tetanus antibody is protective, his pneumococcal titers are below the protective limit in 12 out of 14 serotypes tested.

IgA is the most abundantly produced immunoglobulin and IgA deficiency is usually cited as the most common primary immune deficiency. IgA deficiency is usually diagnosed by complete absence of monomeric IgA in the serum, because the active dimeric form in the mucous membranes is difficult to quantify and is not commercially available.[3-5,18] Most (85%–90%) patients with IgA deficiency are asymptomatic.[5,18] In patients who are symptomatic the deficiency is usually accompanied by gastrointestinal infections, particularly with *Giardia lamblia*, and/or sinopulmonary infections caused by the usual organisms. Celiac disease is reported to occur with higher frequency in IgA-deficient patients, and becomes a diagnostic dilemma because of lack of IgA antibody production; hence, biopsy and human leukocyte antigen testing are necessary for patients who are suspected to have celiac disease and IgA deficiency.[19] Whether or not patients with no serum IgA are at risk for anaphylaxis when receiving blood products because of IgE against IgA is controversial, but most clinicians do warn patients about this possibility.

Autoimmune disease is more common with IgA deficiency, and some of these patients have early common variable immune deficiency (CVID). IgA is usually the first immunoglobulin to fail in CVID.[17] Defects in the transmembrane activator and calcium-modulator and cyclophilin ligand interactor (TACI) protein, encoded by the tumor necrosis factor receptor superfamily member 13B (TNFRSF13B) gene, have been reported in IgA and CVID. It is important to monitor patients with symptomatic IgA deficiency who may have early CVID.[8,17] IgA cannot be replaced, but, if IgG begins to fail, it may be replaced early to avoid serious infection associated with CVID.

Specific antibody deficiency (SAD), previously known as IgG2 subclass deficiency or poor polysaccharide response, is also associated with IgA deficiency.[5,18,20] Poor response to polysaccharide is physiologic early in life (before the age of 2 years) and in the elderly. To counteract the physiologic weaknesses in early and late age, protein conjugate vaccines have been developed, and these are often used in SAD.[8] In extreme cases, IgG replacement is used. The exact diagnostic criteria for this disorder and its treatment remain controversial, but it can also be a harbinger of emerging CVID, and patients with SAD should be monitored for emerging evidence of other deficiencies.[20]

Jimmy receives the rest of his protein conjugate pneumococcal vaccine series and seems to respond (now protected against invasive infection in 12 of 14 serotypes and >1.4 μL/mL in 5 serotypes). He has yearly evaluations with immunoglobulin levels and antibody titers, and within 3 years his pneumococcal serotypes are again below the level of protection in 13 out of 14 serotypes and his IgG level is just below the lower limit for age, which is a change from the previous year. On closer questioning it is revealed that his Aunt Rosalynn has just been diagnosed with CVID and has started IV immunoglobulin.

CVID is a primary immune deficiency that usually is diagnosed in the second or third decade of life.[8] It is now well recognized that CVID is not 1 disorder. There are several genetic defects now identified that may lead to the diagnosis of CVID. The TACI defect has already been discussed. In addition, mutations in the B-cell receptor CD19; the B-cell receptor CD20; the inducible T-cell costimulator, the B cell–activating factor receptor (which is encoded by the TNFRSF13C gene), and mutations in CD81 all have been identified as leading to CVID. Diagnosis of CVID requires a decrease of 2 standard deviations below the norm in IgG and either IgM or IgA levels.[8,21] It also requires evidence of inability to mount an antibody response. Hypogammaglobulinemia itself is not sufficient to diagnose CVID, because other diseases that do not affect antibody production may be responsible for the decrease in immunoglobulin; for example, lymphangiectasia, or nephrotic syndrome.[8] CVID cannot be diagnosed before the age of 4 years because other primary immune deficiencies (including transient hypogammaglobulinemia) must be ruled out.[8] Memory B cells are more frequently lacking in CVID than naive B cells, and the disease is often considered a defect in memory B-cell formation or function, whereas T cells are variably affected.[21]

Presentation is usually increased infection, but particularly in early CVID, diagnosed before or early in the second decade, autoimmune disease may be the initial symptom, although it is often recognized only in retrospect.[22] Autoimmune disease is common in CVID, with immune thrombocytopenia and hemolytic anemia being the most common, and Evans syndrome is a presenting syndrome for many patients with CVID, before infections.[8,17,21,22] Bronchiectasis and granulomatous and lymphocytic interstitial lung disease are two serious lung complications of CVID, the first from chronic infection, the second part of a lymphoproliferative syndrome, a manifestation of inflammation that occurs in 10% to 30% of all patients.[17,21,23] Noninfectious diarrheal disease is one of the most difficult symptoms to control in patients with CVID.[17]

Treatment of CVID includes the use of replacement IgG. One of the major difficulties in effective treatment of CVID is managing necessary immune-suppressive treatment of autoimmune manifestations in patients with a predisposition to infection.

Jimmy has genetic testing that reveals a TACI defect, the same defect found in his Aunt Rosalynn. Over the next 2 years his immunoglobulin level steadily decreases and he is started on replacement-dose subcutaneous immunoglobulin to avoid serious infection. He continues to be monitored closely for any evidence of autoimmune disease and/or infection.

SUMMARY

Humoral immune deficiencies or B-cell deficiencies and defects leading to poor antibody production are the most common primary immune deficiencies, and most manifest in childhood. IgG replacement remains the most important treatment in these patients, who are very susceptible to infection. Because of increasing use of antibiotics, these disorders may come to attention later than would have been true 20 to 30 years ago, but a high index of suspicion allows earlier intervention.

REFERENCES

1. Brambell FW. The transmission of immunity from mother to young and the catabolism of immunoglobulins. Lancet 1966;2:1087–93.

2. Abbas A, Lichtman A, Pillai S. Cellular and molecular immunology. 9th edition. Philadelphia: Elsevier; 2018.

3. Bonilla F, Oettgen H. Adaptive immunity. J Allergy Clin Immunol 2010;125: S33–40.

4. Schroeder H, Cavacini L. Structure and function of immunoglobulins. J Allergy Clin Immunol 2010;125:S41–52.

5. Cunningham-Rundles C. Physiology of IgA and IgA deficiency. J Clin Immunol 2001;21:303–9.

6. Oettegen HC. Regulation of the IgE isotype switch: new insights on cytokine signals and the functions of epsilon germline transcripts. Curr Opin Immunol 2000; 12:618–23.
7. Johansen FE, Brandtzaeg P. Transciptional regulation of the mucosal IgA system. Trends Immunol 2004;25(3):150–7.
8. Bonilla F, Khan DA, Ballas Z, et al. AAAAI practice parameter for the diagnosis and management of primary immune deficiencies. J Allergy Clin Immunol 2015;136(5):1186.
9. Havens PL, Mofenson LM, American Academy of Pediatrics Committee on Pediatric AIDS. Evaluation and management of the infant exposed to HIV-1 in the United States. Pediatrics 2009;123(1):175–87. Available at: http://www.ncbi.nlm.nih.gov/pubmed/19117880.
10. Chan K, Puck JM. Development of population-based newborn screening for severe combined immunodeficiency. J Allergy Clin Immunol 2005;115:391–8.
11. Minegishi Y, Coustan-Smith E, Wang YH, et al. Mutations in the human lambda5/14.1 gene result in B cell deficiency and agammaglobulinemia. J Exp Med 1998; 187:71–7.
12. Yel L, Minegishi Y, Coustan-Smith E, et al. Mutations in the mu heavy chain gene in patients with agammaglobulinemia. N Engl J Med 1996;335:1486–93.
13. Minegishi Y, Coustan-Smith E, Rapalus L, et al. Mutations in Igalpha (CD79a) result in a complete block in B-cell development. J Clin Invest 1999;104:1115–21.
14. Minegishi Y, Rohrer J, Coustan-Smith E, et al. An essential role for BLINK in human B cell development. Science 1999;286:1954–7.
15. Hannarstrin L. Primary Immunodeficiencies screening: neonatal screening for T/B cell disorders-a triplet PCR method for quantification of TRECs and KRECs in newborns. Clin Exp Immunol 2014;178(Suppl1):14–5.
16. Orange J, Hosney E, Weiler C, et al. Use of intravenous immunoglobulin in human disease: a review of evidence by members of the Primary Immunodeficiency Committee of the American Academy of Allergy, Asthma and Immunology 2006;117(4):S525–53. S525–S553.
17. Knight AK, Cunningham-Rundles C. Inflammatory and autoimmune complications of common variable immune deficiency. Autoimmun Rev 2006;5:156–9.
18. Yel L. Selective IgA deficiency. J Clin Immunol 2010;30(1):10–6.
19. Kelly E, Lyon ME, Lyon J, et al. Celiac disease and IgA deficiency: complications of serological testing approaches encountered in the clinic. Clin Chem 2008. https://doi.org/10.1373/clinchem.2008.103606.
20. Perez E, Bonilla F, Orange J, et al. Specific antibody deficiency: controversies in diagnosis and management. Front Immunol 2017;8:586.
21. Filion C, Taylor-Black S, Maglione P, et al. Differentiation of common variable immunodeficiency from IgG deficiency. J Allergy Clin Immunol Pract 2019;7(4): 1277–84.
22. Warrier I, Secord EA. Clinical features of pediatric primary immunodeficiency patients at a tertiary care clinic. AAAAI Conference March 2006, JACI S March 2006.
23. Rao N, Mackinnon AC, Routes J. Granulomatous and Lymphocytic Interstitial Lung Disease (GLILD): a spectrum of pulmonary histopathological lesions in CVID. Hum Pathol 2015;46(9):1306–14.

Innate Immunity

Bani Preet Kaur, MD[a],*, Elizabeth Secord, MD[b]

KEYWORDS

- Innate immunity • Inflammatory response • Immune modulation • Anatomic barriers
- Physiologic barriers • Microbial defense

KEY POINTS

- The innate immune response system forms an important line of defense by deploying a limited number of receptors specific for conserved microbial components.
- A rapid inflammatory response is generated while activating the adaptive immune system.
- Improvements in our understanding of the innate immune system have allowed us to explore various therapeutic strategies via modulation of the immune response.
- Innate immune system encompasses virtually all tissues and involves cells of both hematopoietic and nonhematopoietic origin.

The human microbial defense system can be simplistically viewed as composed of the anatomic and physiologic barriers and the immune response system. The latter has been traditionally divided into 2 branches: adaptive immunity and innate immunity. Adaptive immunity consists of T cell and B cells, with each lymphocyte displaying a specific and structurally unique receptor. This process generates a very large repertoire of antigen receptors thus increasing the probability of encountering an antigen that binds to the given lymphocyte receptor. This process of clonal expansion of lymphocytes does, however, require 3 to 5 days, which could allow the pathogen enough time to cause damage. Innate immunity, composed of phagocytes, antimicrobial peptides, and the complement pathway, constitutes an important first line of defense until a sufficient number of lymphocyte clones are produced and differentiated into effector cells. The innate immune response system targets conserved microbial components shared by a large group of pathogens, generating an inflammatory response within minutes of pathogen exposure. Furthermore, innate immunity plays a key role in triggering the adaptive immune response. In this article, we aim to highlight the basic structure of innate immune system, and expand on its role in human health and disease, especially humoral components and microbial recognition systems.

[a] Detroit Medical Center, Children's Hospital of Michigan, 3901 Beaubien Boulevard, Detroit, MI 48201, USA; [b] Department of Pediatrics, Children's Hospital of Michigan, Wayne State University, 3950 Beaubien Boulevard, Detroit, MI 48202, USA
* Corresponding author.
E-mail address: bani-kaur@uiowa.edu

Pediatr Clin N Am 66 (2019) 905–911
https://doi.org/10.1016/j.pcl.2019.06.011
0031-3955/19/© 2019 Elsevier Inc. All rights reserved.

pediatric.theclinics.com

COMPONENTS OF THE INNATE IMMUNITY

The innate immune system is an evolutionary defense response system with several key features that are shared between different living organisms.[1] It encompasses virtually all tissues and involves cells of both hematopoietic and nonhematopoietic origin. Hematopoietic cells include macrophages, mast cells, neutrophils, eosinophils, dendritic cells and natural killer cells. These cells bear germ line-encoded recognition receptors, become activated during an inflammatory response, and differentiate into short-lived effector cells to rid the infection. Nonhematopoietic components include the skin and epithelial cells lining the gastrointestinal, genitourinary, and respiratory tracts. The commensal microbes in these tissues can become pathogens in case of, for example, a cut or a perforating ulcer. Commensal microbes can also be pathogenic when antibiotics kill most or all microorganisms and overgrowth of the pathogenic microbes occurs. The cellular defenses are further supplemented by humoral components, which include complement proteins, C-reactive protein, lipopolysaccharide (LPS)-binding protein, other pentraxins, collectins, and antimicrobial peptides, including defensins. The circulating proteins of the innate immune system both sense microbes and help with effector mechanisms to facilitate clearance of infection.

INNATE IMMUNE RECOGNITION STRATEGIES AND ACTIVATION OF THE ADAPTIVE IMMUNE SYSTEM

The innate immune response system relies primarily on a limited number of genetically predetermined germ line-encoded receptors that recognize either conserved microbial molecules or common biological sequelae of infections.[2] The problem with predetermined receptor recognition is that every living organism can only encode for a limited number of genes; for example, the human genome has 75,000 to 100,000 genes, most of which are unrelated to immune recognition. In contrast with 10^{18} different T-cell receptors, there are only a few hundred receptors involved in innate immunity and pathogens can mutate at a much higher rate than their hosts. The innate immune system, however, has itself evolved to recognize essential microbial components required for their viability and virulence. What it lacks in variability, the innate immune system makes up by targeting specific nonchanging components of microbes.

The innate immune response system uses 3 primary microbial recognition strategies. The first strategy is to rely on germ line-encoded receptors that are expressed by a large variety of microbes, also known as pattern-recognition receptors. These include the Toll-like receptors (TLRs), NOD-like receptors, C-type lectin receptors, RIG-I–like receptors and AIM2-like receptors. TLRs and C-type lectin receptors are found on the cell surface or on endocytotic compartments. The RIG-I–like receptors, nucleotide oligomerization domain–like receptors (NLRs), and AIM2-like receptors are located in the cytoplasm and survey intracellular pathogens.[3,4] Pattern-recognition receptors recognize highly conserved pathogen-associated molecular patterns (PAMPs), allowing them to distinguish between self-tissues and microbes. PAMPs are only produced by microbes, and are fundamentally integral to the survival and pathogenicity of the microorganisms. Thus, pathogens cannot mutate PAMPs to avoid host immune system detection. Various examples of PAMPs include bacterial membrane components such as endotoxin (LPS), peptidoglycan, mannans, unmethylated microbial DNA, and double-stranded RNA of viral origin.

A second strategy is to identify damage-associated molecular patterns, which represent the metabolic consequence of inflammation and infection. These molecules are upregulated and released during tissue damage and cell lysis during infection and inflammation.[5] Damage-associated molecular patterns include high-mobility group box 1 protein and other endogenous alarmins, heat-shock proteins, and uric acid.

The third approach is to detect missing-self. These are molecules that are expressed by healthy but not infected cells or even microbes. Thus, the recognition of such molecules would indicate normal health thus inhibiting activation of innate immune system against normal host tissue. Natural killer cells are a prime example of this strategy, preferentially attacking only infected cells that downregulate their major histocompatibility complex class I proteins.[6]

The innate immune system, via receptors that are specific for structures found on microbial pathogens, signal the presence of an infection. These signals in turn influence activation of the adaptive immune system. For example, for T-cell activation, 2 signals are required: first, recognition of a ligand in the form of a complex of peptide bound to major histocompatibility complex class II molecule on the surface of an antigen-presenting cell, followed by a costimulatory signal mediated by complement molecules like CD80 and CD86. Receptors like TLRs induce molecules like CD80 and CD86 to appear on antigen-presenting cells following recognition of PAMPs. Although a peptide involved in the peptide–major histocompatibility complex ligand could be a self or microbial peptide, the PAMPs could only occur on pathogens. Thus, TLRs induce CD80 and CD86 only in the presence of an infection thereby ensuring that only pathogen-specific T cells are activated.[7]

TOLL-LIKE RECEPTORS

Drosophila protein Toll was first recognized to be essential in fruit flies for defense against fungal infections in the mid 1990s.[8] The role of TLRs in the innate immune system was then realized when TLR4 (the first human Toll to be characterized) was demonstrated to be a receptor for LPS in mice. Mice with a spontaneous mutation or a targeted disruption of TLR4 gene do not respond to LPS, thus being resistant to endotoxic shock.[9–11] The TLR family consists of 10 receptors, which play a key role in innate immune system.[12] TLRs are involved in the recognition of and response to diverse microbial epitopes, thus allowing discrimination between pathogens and an appropriate cascade of effector adaptive responses.[13] TLRs exist as dimeric proteins (heterodimers or homodimers). The ectodomains of TLRs are composed of leucine-rich repeat motifs, whereas the cytosolic component (Toll/interleukin-receptor) domain is involved in signaling. Individual TLRs recognize a limited number of distinct microbial products; however, collectively the TLR family is able to detect most types of microbial pathogens. TLR signaling pathways allow activation of nuclear factor kappa-B, activator protein-1, interferon-regulatory factor, and other transcription factors, ultimately leading to the production of proinflammatory cytokines, maturation of dendritic cells, and other immunologic responses.

Various human primary immunodeficiencies are associated with abnormal TLR signaling. Monogenic primary immunodeficiencies like IL-1 receptor associated kinase 4 and myeloid differentiation primary response gene 88 deficiencies specifically affect TLR function and pathogen sensing.[14,15] These patients predominantly suffer from recurrent infections caused by pyogenic Gram-positive bacteria, especially *Streptococcus pneumoniae*, as well as *Staphylococcus aureus* and *Pseudomonas aeruginosa*. IL-1 receptor associated kinase 4–deficient patients are, however, resistant to viral infections, which they are able to control via TLR3- and TLR4-dependent production of interferons.[16]

CONTRIBUTION OF TOLL-LIKE RECEPTOR POLYMORPHISMS

A common type of human genetic variation is the single nucleotide polymorphism, where 2 alternative bases occur at appreciable frequency (>1%) in the population.[17] TLR single nucleotide polymorphisms regulate cellular signaling events, cytokine production, and susceptibility to infection based on specific pathogen recognition. Genetic variation involving amino acid changing single nucleotide polymorphisms in TLRs 1, 2, and 5, as well as variants in adaptor molecule Toll/interleukin-receptor domain-containing adaptor protein can result in specific immunodeficiencies. For example, polymorphisms of adaptor molecule MAL/Toll/interleukin-receptor domain-containing adaptor protein, which mediates signaling through TLR 1, 2, 4, and 6 are known to be associated with increased susceptibility to malaria, tuberculosis, and pneumococcal disease.[18] Although several genetic association studies have reported TLR polymorphisms to be associated with susceptibility to infectious and immunologically mediated disease, such results have not been replicated convincingly.

NUCLEOTIDE OLIGOMERIZATION DOMAIN–LIKE RECEPTORS

NLRs are a family of 23 members, structurally divided into N-terminal effector domains.[19] These receptors survey the intracellular environment and sense the microbial products and metabolic stress driving inflammation through the formation of an inflammasome.[20,21] The inflammasome is a large cytoplasmic complex that activates the production of cytokines and inflammatory caspases.[22] The sensing capacity is best demonstrated by NLR family, pyrin domain-containing 3 (NLRP3), which is triggered by metabolic signals like potassium efflux during inflammation owing to plasma membrane disruption or increased extracellular adenosine triphosphate released from injured cells. This activates the caspase-1 inflammasome, leading to IL-1β and IL-18 production.[23]

Cryopyrinopathies are autoinflammatory disorders caused by activating, gain-of-function mutations in NLRP3.[24] The NLRP3 mutations affect IL-1β production, thus leading to IL-1β upregulation. These syndromes include 3 well-described disorders. Familial cold autoinflammatory syndrome (OMIM #120100) manifests as cold-induced fevers, urticaria-like rash, and constitutional symptoms. Muckle-Wells syndrome is characterized by fevers, hives, arthritis, and sensorineural hearing loss unrelated to cold exposure. Finally, neonatal-onset multisystem inflammatory disease (OMIM #607115) is a neonatal disease that presents with urticaria, fever, and chronic aseptic meningitis.[25] These syndromes seem to respond well to the IL-1 receptor antagonist, anakinra.[26]

Studying the NLRs has also shed light on the mechanisms underlying the effects of vaccine adjuvants. Aluminum-containing vaccine adjuvants (alum) serve as immuno-potentiators. It has been demonstrated that the NLRP3 inflammasome is involved in mediating the adjuvant effects of alum through triggering of NLRP3 inflammasome or via release of endogenous signal, uric acid.[27]

IMPLICATIONS OF TOLL-LIKE RECEPTOR ACTIVATION AND MODULATION OF IMMUNE RESPONSE IN ALLERGY AND INFECTIOUS DISEASE

TLR-based therapies specifically target dendritic cell interaction with T cells, a critical component of Th2 immune response associated with allergic inflammation. TLR-based therapies activate dendritic cells, thus producing a cytokine milieu (IL-12, interferons, etc) that favors Th2 immune response inhibition, without directly targeting the T cells.[28]

Studies evaluating modulation of allergic immune responses via TLR activation in preclinical animal models and human participants have primarily studied TLR9 agonists, while some have evaluated TLR4, TLR7/8 agonists. Prior studies have shown that TLR9 agonist CpG DNA inhibits eosinophilic airway inflammation, Th2 cytokine responses, airway remodeling, mucus expression, and airway responsiveness in a mouse model.[29] In humans, the current literature only includes patients with mild asymptomatic asthma, treated with an inhaled TLR9 agonist before allergen challenge.[30] Although this treatment increased expression of IFN-inducible genes, there was neither an inhibition of early or late phase decrease in forced expiratory volume in 1 second nor reduction in sputum eosinophils. Thus, further work is required in this field, testing different doses of TLR9 agonists and different routes of administration or study populations (like symptomatic patients). Likewise, in asymptomatic human participants with ragweed allergic rhinitis, the administration of a topical TLR4 ligand was safe but did not inhibit allergic response to an intranasal ragweed allergen challenge.[31] No human studies in allergy or asthma have been reported with a TLR7/8 agonist.

Previous studies have evaluated whether a TLR9 agonist conjugated to an allergen would enhance its immunogenicity. Studies in mouse models have shown a 100-fold enhanced uptake of TLR9-conjugated allergen by an antigen-presenting cell compared with TLR9 ligand alone. This is accompanied by a 100-fold greater induction in Th1 immune response than equivalent amounts of a nonconjugated mixture of TLR9 ligand and allergen.[28]

However, studies in humans evaluating the effectiveness of TLR9 ragweed allergen vaccine have produced conflicting results. A Canadian study in patients with ragweed allergic rhinitis demonstrated a decrease in nasal mucosal biopsy eosinophil counts and Th2 cytokines after the administration of the TLR9 ragweed allergen vaccine, but no decrease in nasal symptom scores during the ragweed season.[32] Another study demonstrated a significant decrease in rhinitis symptom scores after the administration of TLR9 ragweed allergy vaccine in patients with ragweed-induced allergic rhinitis during ragweed season. Furthermore, there was a decrease in doses of allergy rescue medications in these participants. Interestingly, the benefit of symptom reduction was noted to persist into the second ragweed season without any additional vaccine.[33]

The immunologic mechanisms underlying the success of vaccines in preventing infectious diseases are unclear. Subunit vaccines, in contrast with live vaccines, require adjuvant supplementation to augment their immunogenicity and thus promote a protective immune response. However, there is a paucity of licensed safe and effective adjuvants for clinical use. The understanding of innate immune system biology (eg, mechanism of action of alum adjuvancy in the NLR system) has initiated development of novel vaccine adjuvants.[34] Monophosphoryl lipid A (MPL) is one such example that comes from the cell wall LPS of gram-negative *Salmonella* Minnesota R595 and is detoxified.[35] MPL retains adjuvant properties without the toxicity of LPS. MPL combined with aluminum salt has been efficacious in vaccines against human papilloma virus and hepatitis B. This combination uses both TLR pathway (triggered by MPL) and NALP3 inflammasome (alum crystals) to promote an immune response.

SUMMARY

The innate immune response system forms an important line of defense by deploying a limited number of receptors specific for conserved microbial components. This generates a rapid inflammatory response, while activating the adaptive immune system.

Improvements in our understanding of the innate immune system have allowed us to explore various therapeutic strategies via modulation of the immune response.

REFERENCES

1. Turvey SE, Broide DH. Innate immunity. J Allergy Clin Immunol 2010; 125(2 Suppl 2):S24–32.
2. Janeway CA Jr, Medzhitov R. Innate immune recognition. Annu Rev Immunol 2002;20:197–216.
3. Janeway CA Jr. Approaching the asymptote? Evolution and revolution in immunology. Cold Spring Harb Symp Quant Biol 1989;54 Pt 1:1–13.
4. Brubaker SW, Bonham KS, Zanoni I, et al. Innate immune pattern recognition: a cell biological perspective. Annu Rev Immunol 2015;33:257–90.
5. Bianchi ME. DAMPs, PAMPs and alarmins: all we need to know about danger. J Leukoc Biol 2007;81(1):1–5.
6. Joncker NT, Raulet DH. Regulation of NK cell responsiveness to achieve self-tolerance and maximal responses to diseased target cells. Immunol Rev 2008; 224:85–97.
7. Medzhitov R, Janeway C Jr. Innate immunity. N Engl J Med 2000;343(5):338–44.
8. Lemaitre B, Nicolas E, Michaut L, et al. The dorsoventral regulatory gene cassette spatzle/Toll/cactus controls the potent antifungal response in Drosophila adults. Cell 1996;86(6):973–83.
9. Poltorak A, He X, Smirnova I, et al. Defective LPS signaling in C3H/HeJ and C57BL/10ScCr mice: mutations in Tlr4 gene. Science 1998;282(5396):2085–8.
10. Qureshi ST, Lariviere L, Leveque G, et al. Endotoxin-tolerant mice have mutations in Toll-like receptor 4 (Tlr4). J Exp Med 1999;189(4):615–25.
11. Hoshino K, Takeuchi O, Kawai T, et al. Cutting edge: toll-like receptor 4 (TLR4)-deficient mice are hyporesponsive to lipopolysaccharide: evidence for TLR4 as the Lps gene product. J Immunol 1999;162(7):3749–52.
12. Takeda K, Kaisho T, Akira S. Toll-like receptors. Annu Rev Immunol 2003;21: 335–76.
13. Akira S, Takeda K. Toll-like receptor signalling. Nat Rev Immunol 2004;4(7): 499–511.
14. Picard C, Puel A, Bonnet M, et al. Pyogenic bacterial infections in humans with IRAK-4 deficiency. Science 2003;299(5615):2076–9.
15. von Bernuth H, Picard C, Jin Z, et al. Pyogenic bacterial infections in humans with MyD88 deficiency. Science 2008;321(5889):691–6.
16. Yang K, Puel A, Zhang S, et al. Human TLR-7-, -8-, and -9-mediated induction of IFN-alpha/beta and -lambda Is IRAK-4 dependent and redundant for protective immunity to viruses. Immunity 2005;23(5):465–78.
17. Goldstein DB, Cavalleri GL. Genomics: understanding human diversity. Nature 2005;437(7063):1241–2.
18. Khor CC, Chapman SJ, Vannberg FO, et al. A Mal functional variant is associated with protection against invasive pneumococcal disease, bacteremia, malaria and tuberculosis. Nat Genet 2007;39(4):523–8.
19. Ting JP, Lovering RC, Alnemri ES, et al. The NLR gene family: a standard nomenclature. Immunity 2008;28(3):285–7.
20. Chen G, Shaw MH, Kim YG, et al. NOD-like receptors: role in innate immunity and inflammatory disease. Annu Rev Pathol 2009;4:365–98.
21. Benko S, Philpott DJ, Girardin SE. The microbial and danger signals that activate Nod-like receptors. Cytokine 2008;43(3):368–73.

22. Martinon F, Mayor A, Tschopp J. The inflammasomes: guardians of the body. Annu Rev Immunol 2009;27:229–65.
23. Franchi L, Eigenbrod T, Munoz-Planillo R, et al. The inflammasome: a caspase-1-activation platform that regulates immune responses and disease pathogenesis. Nat Immunol 2009;10(3):241–7.
24. Masters SL, Simon A, Aksentijevich I, et al. Horror autoinflammaticus: the molecular pathophysiology of autoinflammatory disease (*). Annu Rev Immunol 2009; 27:621–68.
25. Aksentijevich I, Nowak M, Mallah M, et al. De novo CIAS1 mutations, cytokine activation, and evidence for genetic heterogeneity in patients with neonatal-onset multisystem inflammatory disease (NOMID): a new member of the expanding family of pyrin-associated autoinflammatory diseases. Arthritis Rheum 2002; 46(12):3340–8.
26. Goldbach-Mansky R, Dailey NJ, Canna SW, et al. Neonatal-onset multisystem inflammatory disease responsive to interleukin-1beta inhibition. N Engl J Med 2006; 355(6):581–92.
27. Eisenbarth SC, Colegio OR, O'Connor W, et al. Crucial role for the Nalp3 inflammasome in the immunostimulatory properties of aluminium adjuvants. Nature 2008;453(7198):1122–6.
28. Horner AA, Redecke V, Raz E. Toll-like receptor ligands: hygiene, atopy and therapeutic implications. Curr Opin Allergy Clin Immunol 2004;4(6):555–61.
29. Broide D, Schwarze J, Tighe H, et al. Immunostimulatory DNA sequences inhibit IL-5, eosinophilic inflammation, and airway hyperresponsiveness in mice. J Immunol 1998;161(12):7054–62.
30. Gauvreau GM, Hessel EM, Boulet LP, et al. Immunostimulatory sequences regulate interferon-inducible genes but not allergic airway responses. Am J Respir Crit Care Med 2006;174(1):15–20.
31. Casale TB, Kessler J, Romero FA. Safety of the intranasal toll-like receptor 4 agonist CRX-675 in allergic rhinitis. Ann Allergy Asthma Immunol 2006;97(4): 454–6.
32. Tulic MK, Fiset PO, Christodoulopoulos P, et al. Amb a 1-immunostimulatory oligodeoxynucleotide conjugate immunotherapy decreases the nasal inflammatory response. J Allergy Clin Immunol 2004;113(2):235–41.
33. Creticos PS, Schroeder JT, Hamilton RG, et al. Immunotherapy with a ragweed-toll-like receptor 9 agonist vaccine for allergic rhinitis. N Engl J Med 2006; 355(14):1445–55.
34. Pulendran B, Ahmed R. Translating innate immunity into immunological memory: implications for vaccine development. Cell 2006;124(4):849–63.
35. Casella CR, Mitchell TC. Putting endotoxin to work for us: monophosphoryl lipid A as a safe and effective vaccine adjuvant. Cell Mol Life Sci 2008;65(20):3231–40.

Newborn Screening for Severe Combined Immunodeficiency

Mohammed Taki, MD[a], Tayaba Miah, MD[a],
Elizabeth Secord, MD[b],*

KEYWORDS

- Severe combined immunodeficiency (SCID) • T-cell receptor excision circle (tREC)
- Newborn screening (NBS) • T-cell lymphopenia

KEY POINTS

- The T-cell receptor excision circle (TREC) assay is an effective screening tool for severe combined immunodeficiency (SCID).
- The TREC assay was designed to detect typical SCID and leaky SCID, but any condition causing low naïve T-cell counts will also be detected.
- Newborn screening for SCID using the TREC assay has proven itself to be highly sensitive and cost-efficient. This review covers the history of SCID newborn screening, elaborates on the SCID subtypes and TREC assay limitations, and discusses diagnostic and management considerations for infants with a positive screen.

INTRODUCTION

Severe combined immunodeficiency (SCID) is a syndrome caused by defects in genes responsible for orchestrating the maturation of elements of the adaptive immune system. SCID is genetically heterogeneous (mutations in >20 genes have been identified), but all forms result in a marked decrease in naïve T cells, and subsequently impaired cellular and humoral immunity. Infants are left at risk for recurrent severe infections, chronic diarrhea, and failure to thrive. Infants with SCID appear normal at birth, and maternal antibodies provide some measure of protection until they wane around 4 to 6 months of age. Untreated, SCID patients are expected to succumb to recurrent and opportunistic infections by 2 years of age.[1,2]

Before the advent of newborn screening (NBS) for SCID, most patients were identified after presenting with clinical symptoms or were identified by family history.

Disclosure Statement: The authors have nothing to disclose.
[a] Department of Pediatrics, Children's Hospital of Michigan, 3901 Beaubien Street, Detroit, MI 48201, USA; [b] Department of Allergy and Immunology, Children's Hospital of Michigan, 3901 Beaubien Street, Detroit, MI 48201, USA
* Corresponding author. Department of Pediatrics, Children's Hospital of Michigan, Wayne State University, 3950 Beaubien Boulevard, Detroit, MI 48202.
E-mail address: Ae8701@wayne.edu

Shortening this delay in diagnosis was critical, because affected infants can be successfully treated with hematopoietic stem cell transplantation, gene therapy, or enzyme replacement therapy (for adenosine deaminase deficiency) provided they are diagnosed before infections become overwhelming.[3–6] T-cell receptor excision circles (TRECs) are an indicator of T-cell lymphopoiesis, and quantitative polymerase chain reaction (PCR) measurement of this biomarker is an effective screening test for SCID, regardless of the underlying genetic cause.[7] In 2008, Wisconsin became the first state to implement NBS for SCID using the TREC assay. After subsequent review, the US Secretary of Health and Human Services added SCID to the Recommended Uniform Screening Panel (RUSP) in 2010. As of December 2018, all 50 states have added SCID to their NBS programs.[8,9]

This review covers current screening assays for SCID with a brief historical explanation of SCID NBS, elaborates on assay limitations and SCID subtypes, and discusses diagnostic and management considerations for infants with a positive screen.

HISTORY OF SEVERE COMBINED IMMUNODEFICIENCY NEWBORN SCREENING

In the United States, NBS programs run at the state level began in the 1960s with the development of a filter paper–based system, onto which newborns' heel-stick blood samples were spotted and dried. Robert Guthrie's innovation, spurred by his experience with his son and niece experiencing neurodevelopmental delays from phenylketonuria (PKU), provided blood samples that were easy to obtain and stable. His assay for PKU was accurate, consistent, and inexpensive, providing the paradigm for future NBS assays.[4] Because early intervention before the onset of symptoms from PKU is effective, this disease also exemplified the types of disorders that would benefit from NBS programs. In 1968, Wilson and Jungner[5] suggested specific criteria for the addition of diseases to NBS programs, which continue to inform discussions about population-based screening. Judged by these criteria, SCID is an excellent target for NBS. It is a life-threatening health problem; treatment is available and most effective in the latent presymptomatic stage, and natural history of SCID is well understood. Identification of at-risk infants before the onset of severe and life-threatening infections would decrease the morbidity and mortality associated with these disorders.

NBS programs represent a complex system of screening, education, follow-up, diagnosis, evaluation, and treatment/management that must be implemented within state governments. The development of such a system will inevitably be influenced by economic, political, and cultural factors. All acceptable screening assays must be sensitive and specific, widely available, reproducible, and affordable. In the 1970s, attempts to screen for adenosine deaminase (ADA)-deficiency, a subtype of SCID, were unsuccessful because of insufficient sensitivity and specificity of the enzyme assay used.[6,10,11] Immunoassays detecting either interleukin7, which induces proliferation and differentiation of thymocytes, or CD3 and CD45, cell markers for T cells and lymphocytes, respectively, were proposed but never developed into robust assays.[12,13] Another approach was to screen DNA from the dried blood spot samples for mutations in known SCID disease genes. Although this method could screen for both known disease-causing mutations as well as detect previously unreported sequence variants likely to cause disease, there are hundreds of mutations described in the known genes, with more being discovered. To compound the problem, there are cases of SCID whereby no mutation has been identified despite extensive DNA sequencing.[14,15] Relying on DNA screening would introduce an unacceptable rate of false negatives. There is a high degree of variation in the underlying genetics, yet all SCID is characterized by decreased or absent naïve T cells. To exploit this principle, investigators explored lymphocyte profiles as the next target. This method screened for absolute lymphocyte counts. The main limitation of this approach was the high degree of overlap in lymphocyte counts between some forms of SCID and healthy infants. No adequate threshold could be found to optimize the rate of false negatives versus false positives. Furthermore, this method required liquid blood samples (umbilical cord blood was also attempted), which posed significant financial and logistical barriers when compared with a dry blood spot assay.[16,17]

THE T-CELL RECEPTOR EXCISION CIRCLE ASSAY FOR SEVERE COMBINED IMMUNODEFICIENCY

T lymphocytes' ability to provide adequate defense against a diverse repertoire of pathogens requires an equally diverse range of T-cell receptors (TCR). Recombination of a large number of gene loci organized into segments, known as variable (V), diversity (D), and joining (J) regions. These genes code for TCR chains (and antibody molecules) and lie near genes coding for constant regions. During TCR rearrangement, a series of enzymes introduce double-stranded DNA breaks at specific sites, rejoin different segments, and then process and repair the segments. The excised DNA fragments, which are not incorporated into the TCR, can form a variety of circular DNA structures known as TRECs.[18] Approximately 70% to 80% of thymocytes will ultimately produce 1 specific TREC known as the δRec-ψJa TREC.[19,20] A quantitative PCR can then be used to provide a TREC copy number, an indicator of naïve T cells migrating from the thymus into peripheral circulation (**Fig. 1**).[21]

Crucially, TRECs are not produced when mature T cells divide, making them selective for newly produced naïve T cells.[22] Consequently, the SCID assay has excellent sensitivity and specificity for SCID, including some situations where infants may have near normal T-cell numbers (leaky SCID, maternal lymphocyte engraftment). Chan and Puck[21] published the first method for SCID screening using PCR to obtain TREC measurements from dried blood spots in 2005. The assay also involved the amplification of a control gene (β-actin) to differentiate between samples with low TREC levels owing to truly low levels of naïve T cells and those with low TREC levels owing to degradation of DNA or poor sample quality.[21] A TREC assay is only considered positive when a sample has low levels of TRECs, but normal levels of control gene. Whether the control PCR is performed simultaneously with the TREC PCR, or only on samples with low levels of TRECs, varies by state.

In the United States, the federal government publishes the RUSP, a list of recommended diseases to be included in NBS screening programs. The final decision to add a disease to NBS programs is made by individual states, however. Wisconsin was the first state to introduce NBS for SCID using the TREC assay in 2008.[8] The data from this program established the TREC assay as a viable NBS method. After reviewing these results, the Secretary's Advisory Committee on Heritable Disorders in Newborns and Children unanimously recommended adding SCID to the RUSP.[9] In 2010, the Secretary of Health and Human Services accepted this recommendation and formally added SCID to the RUSP. States began to accelerate the rate of implementation of SCID screening into their NBS programs. As of December 2018, all 50 states screen newborns for SCID.[23]

SEVERE COMBINED IMMUNODEFICIENCY SUBTYPES AND OTHER CONDITIONS DETECTED BY T-CELL RECEPTOR EXCISION CIRCLES ASSAY

The TRECs assay was designed to detect typical SCID and leaky SCID, but any condition causing low naïve T-cell counts will also be detected. Typical SCID is diagnosed

TCRA locus

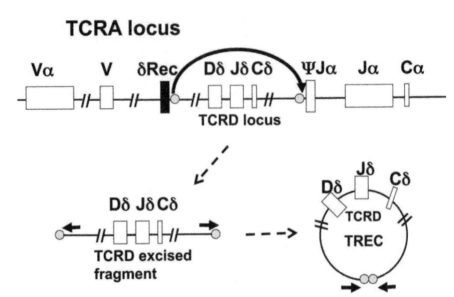

Fig. 1. Generation of the δRec-ψJα TRECs. The germline configuration of the TCRA locus, with TCRD embedded, is shown at the top of the illustration, which also shows the points (*gray dots*) at which the DNA is cut to excise the TCRD locus in T-lymphocyte progenitors destined to express the α and β TCRs. After excision (*lower left*) and ligation (*lower right*) of the δRec-ψJα fragment to form a TREC, PCR primers (*horizontal arrows*) can amplify a DNA junction fragment containing the joint. (*From* Kwan, A., MBBS, PhD, & Puck, J., MD. (2015). History and current status of newborn screening for severe combined immunodeficiency. Seminars in Perinatology, 39, 194-205. doi:https://doi.org/10.1053/j.semperi.2015.03.004.)

when there are less than 300 T cells/μL and less than 10% of normal T-cell proliferation on phytohemagglutinin mitogen proliferation culture.[24] Frequently, these patients will also exhibit maternal T-cell engraftment owing to survival of maternal T cells that have crossed transplacentally. These cells would normally be eliminated by immune competent T cells in healthy newborns. Typical SCID is also the most likely to be associated with mutations in known SCID genes. Leaky SCID is defined as T-cell counts between 300 and 1499/μL (perhaps higher if oligoclonal lines are present), reduced proliferation on PHA mitogen culture, no maternal engraftment, and an incomplete or hypomorphic (partial loss of function) mutation in SCID genes. Generally, the mutations causing leaky SCID result in a product that has abnormal, but not absent, function. Omenn syndrome has similar findings to leaky SCID and also includes oligoclonal T-cell lines, erythroderma, elevated eosinophil and immunoglobulin E (IgE) levels, and hepatosplenomegaly.[25] Other syndromes that are associated with low naïve T cells may be detected by the TRECs assay, including DiGeorge syndrome, trisomy 21, CHARGE syndrome, and ataxia telangiectasia.[26] Secondary causes of T-cell lymphopenia, such as cardiac defects, gastrointestinal abnormalities, or multiple congenital defects, may also be detected by the TRECs assay.[27] The lymphopenia in these cases is most frequently caused by shifting of T lymphocytes from intravascular to extravascular space, with no intrinsic defect in T lymphopoiesis. Finally, some patients have low T-cell numbers with unclear cause, an entity known as idiopathic T-cell lymphopenia, or variant SCID.

Furthermore, the TREC assay has limitations in its ability to identify disorders characterized by impaired T-cell function, leading to false negative results. For instance, in infants with ADA-deficient SCID, maternal detoxification of elevated levels of purine intermediates in utero allows for temporary protection of fetal T cell, which can sometimes yield normal birth TREC levels. However, TREC and T-cell numbers eventually drop, leading to a delayed- or late-onset of ADA-SCID, which may have been missed on the initial NBS.[10,11] In addition, in some genetic defects that affect the development of the T cell after VDJ recombination, such as in ZAP-70 (zeta chain–associated protein kinase-70) deficiency, TREC assays may yield a false negative result despite functionally incompetent T cells. Although TREC assay can detect some immunodeficiencies in addition to SCID as discussed previously, it does have its limitations in detecting various other primary immunodeficiencies. Some examples of conditions undetectable by the assay include CD40 ligand deficiency, major histocompatibility complex class II deficiency, primary immunodeficiencies limited to B cells and humoral immunity, and combined immune deficiencies with low, but not absent T-cell function.[28,29]

RESULTS OF SEVERE COMBINED IMMUNODEFICIENCY NEWBORN SCREENING

Kwan and colleagues[30] published the early results of SCID NBS for more than 3 million infants (n = 3,030,083) from programs in the first 10 states to offer screening, and the Navajo nation. The states included were California, Colorado, Connecticut, Delaware, Massachusetts, Michigan, Mississippi, New York, Texas, and Wisconsin. All programs used the TRECs assay to screen newborns; positive assays were confirmed with flow cytometry to definitively determine T-, B-, and NK-lymphocyte numbers, and enumerate naïve versus memory T cells. Different states used different TREC threshold values to trigger flow cytometry screening, resulting in variation in number of referrals. The precise cutoff defining "T-cell lymphopenia" also resulted in varying rates of false positive results, which in this case means low TREC counts referred for flow cytometry that subsequently shows T cells above chosen cutoff for "T-cell lymphopenia." The false positive rate ranged from 0% to 82%.

The results of all states averaged showed 1.72 cases of SCID per 100,000 infants screened (95% confidence interval 1.3–2.2). The overall incidence of SCID was found to be 1 in 58,000 live births with no statistically significant difference between states. As expected, the Navajo Nation did have a higher incidence of 1 in 3500 births, because of a widespread founder mutation in a DNA repair protein. Previous studies have estimated SCID incidence in this population to be 1 in 2000 births. Overall, 52 cases of SCID were diagnosed, which includes 9 individuals with leaky SCID and 1 individual with Omenn syndrome. No cases of SCID were missed and later diagnosed.[30]

Of the 42 infants identified as having typical SCID, 9 were found to have mutations in *IL2RG* gene, which codes for the common γ chain of the cytokine receptor. Six infants had typical SCID from mutations in IL7RA, and 5 infants had adenosine deaminase deficiency, which leads to impairment in purine metabolism and accumulation of toxic metabolites. Mutations in the Recombinase activating gene 1 (RAG1), which lead to dysfunction of V(D)J recombination, were found in 4 infants. Janus kinase 3 (JAK3) mutation accounted for 3 of the infants with typical SCID. The following mutations accounted for 1 case each: DCLRE1 C, RAG2, CD3D, TC7A, and Pallister-Killian syndrome with tetrasomy 12p.[30] Six infants had no mutation identified after all typical mutations associated with SCID were ruled out. Mutations tested were for genes coding for the common γ chain, interleukin-7 receptor, recombinase activating genes, adenosine deaminase, purine nucleoside phosphorylase, JAK3, Artemis, and CD3 receptor complex. The remaining 4 patients did not have genetic testing completed. Of the 10 leaky SCID cases, 4 infants had RAG1 mutations, 2 were found to have RMRP mutation, and 1 each had mutations in IL2RG and DCLRE1 C, respectively. The remaining 2 infants had no mutation found after all typical SCID-associated genes were ruled out.[30]

This study also reported 411 infants identified as having T-cell lymphopenia that was not related to SCID. Approximately one-third had syndromes with T-cell impairment (n = 136/411); another 28% had secondary T-cell impairment (n = 117/411), and 7% had T-cell lymphopenia associated with preterm birth alone. Twelve were diagnosed with variant SCID (which had hematopoietic stem cell transplant performed). An additional 28% (n = 117/411) had unspecified T-cell lymphopenia, with no further information available at the time of publication, although at least in 1 state these patients were undergoing monitoring and treatment of T-cell deficiency.[30]

EVALUATION OF INFANTS WITH POSITIVE T-CELL RECEPTOR EXCISION CIRCLES RESULTS

The protocol for evaluating infants with positive (low) TREC results on NBS varies by state.[31] Results are not considered abnormal if numbers of both TRECs and β-actin are found to be low, because this would indicate degradation of the DNA sample as opposed to true T-cell lymphopenia. Some states have protocols that will repeat the TREC assay on premature infants, which are known to more frequently have low TRECs despite no intrinsic defect in T-cell production, until these infants reach a corrected gestational age of at least 36 weeks. In several states, the results of abnormal TREC assays are reported to the infant's primary care doctor as well as to a clinical immunologist.[32] These physicians, once notified, work with families to evaluate the infants further.

The results of the TREC assay as well as the clinical history of the infant will guide the evaluation. The TREC assay results are reported as absolute values, which will inform the level of urgency required. Infants having severely decreased TREC values are at higher risk for having SCID and thus require urgent evaluation. Communicating with the primary care provider or the family is also paramount. The immunologist should determine if there were any conditions in the prenatal or postnatal period that may have contributed to an abnormal TREC screening. Prenatal issues include infections or medications the mother took during pregnancy. Premature birth as well as infections or congenital anomalies may affect the TREC assay.[33] If there are medical conditions that can be treated, it may be prudent to postpone the full immunologic workup until these conditions are treated, or to repeat after treatment. Immunologists should be aware of the protocol used in her or his state, because not all states repeat TREC assays in premature infants.

Flow cytometry to enumerate lymphocyte numbers is the initial study used in the evaluation of infants with abnormal TREC results. This study will provide the numbers of T cells, B cells, and NK cells and must also provide the percentage of naïve (CD45RA$^+$) versus memory (CD45RO$^+$) T cells present.[34] T-lymphocytes of maternal origin will be memory cells and flow cytometry will therefore identify maternal engraftment. Normal neonate T cells are approximately 90% naïve.[35] Flow cytometry provides the initial confirmatory diagnostic test after TREC screening. If T-lymphocyte numbers are normal, then no further workup is required. Infants who show decreased T lymphocytes, or a preponderance of memory T lymphocytes, will require further evaluation by the immunologist.

Abnormal results on the above studies will indicate possible SCID or leaky SCID. These infants should be hospitalized in a single room, and any sick contacts prohibited, or kept at home with strict precautions if hospitalization is not possible due to hospital policy/insurance barriers. Most centers now encourage hospitalization in protective isolation if at all possible. Any clinical abnormalities, including respiratory distress, signs of infection, or autoimmune conditions, should be diagnosed and treated. The patient and family should avoid live vaccinations, including rotavirus vaccine, and all family members should be vaccinated against influenza. Mothers should be advised to stop breastfeeding until maternal cytomegalovirus (CMV) exposure is assessed with CMV IgG serology. Seropositive mothers should avoid nursing, and infant CMV PCR should be checked weekly for 4 weeks, and periodically thereafter.[36] Nutritional support should be provided, and infants should be monitored for iron deficiency. A social worker should be introduced to the family to help with support and services. Immunoglobulins should be administered to maintain IgG levels greater than 800 mg/dL. Palivizumab may be administered during the respiratory syncytial virus season.[33] Prophylactic antimicrobials should be initiated, including fluconazole, acyclovir, and trimethoprim-sulfamethoxazole after 30 days of life. Human leukocyte antigen typing should be performed on parents and siblings to evaluate as potential donors for hematopoietic stem cell transplant. If there is no match, a search for matching an unrelated individual must be initiated.[37]

Early clinical and laboratory assessment of infants with suspected SCID should include a detailed history, including infections, diarrhea, or failure to thrive. Family history, including immune deficiencies and early childhood deaths, should be obtained. Pedigree analysis and history of consanguinity should be ascertained. Physical examination should document any dysmorphic features, signs of infection, presence of tonsils and other lymphoid tissues, cardiac abnormalities, and rash or erythroderma. Families should be counseled on infection prevention precautions: avoidance of sick contacts and public places, use of boiled water exclusively, no well water, withholding breast-feeding until maternal CMV status is known, avoidance of live vaccinations, and the use of irradiated and CMV-negative blood products (should any be required). Infants should have PCR or antigen detection assays for respiratory viruses, adenovirus, rotavirus, human immunodeficiency virus, herpes simplex virus, Epstein-Barr virus, hepatitis B, and parvovirus B19. Quantitative immunoglobulins should be checked before administration of intravenous immunoglobulin, including IgG, IgA, IgM, and IgE. Lymphocyte proliferation assay to phytohemagglutinin, if not already done, should be performed. Note that a larger-than-usual blood sample may be required to account for low lymphocyte numbers; in addition, the laboratory should be informed of the low T-cell count before running the sample.[33,36] Adenosine deaminase and purine nucleoside phosphorylase levels should be obtained, unless family history strongly suggests a different genotype of SCID. DNA sequencing targeting known genetic causes of SCID should be sent.[36–38] Infant gender and lymphocyte profile (whether B cells and NK cells are present) may direct the molecular diagnosis. If there is a suspected genotype, the specific gene may be sequenced first; otherwise, a panel of SCID genes should be sequenced.[39] Establishing a genetic diagnosis will help guide further management. Certain subtypes of SCID, usually caused by defects in DNA repair mechanisms, can be sensitive to radiation. These subtypes include deficiencies of Artemis, DNA Ligase IV, DNA-dependent protein kinase catalytic subunit, Cernunnos-XLF, and nibrin.[40] DNA sequencing or Western blotting for LIG4 and NHEJ should be done. If these genotypes are ruled out, a chest radiograph should be obtained to evaluate whether a thymus is visible; evaluating the lung parenchyma and osseous structures is also helpful.

Infants with acute illnesses, congenital syndromes, or conditions associated with T-cell lymphopenia must be followed longitudinally. These infants should have repeat flow cytometry when they are clinically stable, and T-lymphocyte numbers should be followed to ensure they normalize. These patients will also benefit from immunoglobulin levels and antibody recall titers. Infants with multiple congenital anomalies or dysmorphic features should undergo genetic studies for deletions and duplications.

A genetic diagnosis is not required before proceeding with hematopoietic stem cell transplantation. This decision is made based on the infant's clinical picture and immunologic findings. Infants with adenosine deaminase deficiency may be treated with enzyme replacement therapy, before stem cell transplant. The prognosis for infants diagnosed with SCID or leaky SCID on NBS has been promising. Hematopoietic stem cell transplantation in infants with no infections has resulted in 2-year survival rates of approximately 95%. Infants with infections have a survival rate of around 81%.[41,42] Gene therapy for known genetic causes of SCID is expected to be an option in the future.

SUMMARY

The TRECs assay is an effective screening tool for SCID. TREC numbers are an indication of naïve T cells, which have recently migrated from the thymus. It follows that the TREC assay detects T-cell lymphopenia from any cause. Most infants with positive TRECs assays do not have SCID (approximately 90%, according to 1 study).[30] Congenital syndromes and secondary causes of T-cell lymphopenia are the most common cause of low TREC numbers on NBS. Complete or severe DiGeorge syndrome is the most common primary immunodeficiency detected by the TREC assay, but the assay does not detect all infants with DiGeorge, only those with very low T cells. Other combined immunodeficiencies that have variability in number of naïve T cells will not be detected by the TRECs assay. Clinicians should be aware of these limitations and not have a false sense of security. Clinical judgment must be used when evaluating infants for primary immunodeficiencies, regardless of the results of NBS.

NBS for SCID using the TRECs assay has proven itself to be effective and cost-efficient. Most infants born in the United States are currently screened for SCID.[23] Results of NBS for SCID so far show an overall incidence of 1 in 58,000.[30] The TRECs assay has been shown to have a predictive value for T-cell lymphopenia of approximately 50% and has sensitivity of nearly 100% for diagnosis of SCID and leaky SCID.[23] Infants with SCID identified on NBS have an excellent prognosis following hematopoietic stem cell transplantation.

NBS with the TRECs assay has brought increased attention to a subset of patients with idiopathic T-cell lymphopenia. The management of such infants is not clearly defined, and further research is needed to provide guidance on the appropriate level of monitoring and intervention in these infants. The laboratory evaluation of infants with positive TRECs assay, including flow cytometry, lymphocyte proliferation assays, and genetic testing, is not available in all areas, and there are many immunologists with the expertise to diagnose and treat SCID and other severe primary immunodeficiencies. Obtaining genetic testing to establish a clear diagnosis is not straightforward in many states, and there are significant insurance barriers in some cases. Outreach programs to educate primary care physicians and families about SCID NBS would be beneficial. SCID NBS using the TREC assay represents an important advance in the early diagnosis of SCID and other forms of T-cell lymphopenia. For hundreds of infants and families in the United States, these efforts represent a chance at a longer, healthier life.

REFERENCES

1. van der Burg M, Gennery AR. Educational paper. The expanding clinical and immunological spectrum of severe combined immunodeficiency. Eur J Pediatr 2011;170:561.
2. Notarangelo LD. Primary immunodeficiencies. J Allergy Clin Immunol 2010;125: S182–94.
3. Myers LA, Patel DD, Puck JM, et al. Hematopoietic stem cell transplantation for severe combined immunodeficiency in the neonatal period leads to superior thymic output and improved survival. Blood 2002;99(3):872–8.
4. Centerwall WR, Chinnock RF, Pusavat A. Phenylketonuria: screening programs and testing methods. Am J Public Health 1960;50(11):1667–77.
5. Wilson JM, Jungner YG. Principles and Practice of Screening for Disease. Public health papers, vol. 34, 1968. p. 7–151. Geneva (Switzerland). Available at: http://www.who.int/iris/handle/10665/37650. Accessed July 20, 2019.
6. Kalman L, Lindegren ML, Kobrynski L, et al. Mutations in genes required for T-cell development:IL7R,CD45,IL2RG, JAK3, RAG1,RAG2,ARTEMIS,and ADA and severe combined immunodeficiency: HuGE review. GenetMed 2004;6(1):16–26.
7. Accetta Pedersen DJ, Verbsky J, Routes JM. Screening newborns for primary T-cell immunodeficiencies: consensus and controversy. Expert Rev Clin Immunol 2011;7:761–8.
8. Baker MW, Grossman WJ, Laessig RH, et al. Development of a routine newborn screening protocol for severe combined immunodeficiency. J Allergy Clin Immunol 2009;124:8272–9.
9. Routes JM, Grossman WJ, Verbsky J, et al. Statewide newborn screening for severe T-cell lymphopenia. JAMA 2009;302:2465–70.
10. Moore EC, Meuwissen HJ. Screening for ADA deficiency. J Pediatr 1974;85(6): 802–4.
11. Hirschhorn R. Adenosine deaminase deficiency. Immunodefic Rev 1990;2(3): 175–98.
12. Bolotin E, Annett G, Parkman R, et al. Serum levels of IL-7 in bone marrow transplant recipients: relationship to clinical characteristics and lymphocyte count. Bone Marrow Transplant 1999;23(8):783–8.
13. McGhee SA, Stiehm ER, Cowan M, et al. Two-tiered universal newborn screening strategy for severe combined immunodeficiency. Mol Genet Metab 2005;86(4): 427–30.
14. Lebet T, Chiles R, Hsu AP, et al. Mutations causing severe combined immunodeficiency: detection with a custom resequencing microarray. Genet Med 2008; 10(8):575–85.
15. Puck JM. Laboratory technology for population-based screening for severe combined immunodeficiency in neonates: the winner is T-cell receptor excision circles. J Allergy Clin Immunol 2012;129(3):607–16.
16. Collier F, Tang M, Ponsonby AL, et al. Flow cytometric assessment of cord blood as an alternative strategy for population-based screening of severe combined immunodeficiency. J Allergy Clin Immunol 2013;131(4):1251–2.
17. de Villartay JP. V(D)J recombination deficiencies. Adv Exp Med Biol 2009;650: 46–58.
18. Morinishi Y, Imai K, Nakagawa N, et al. Identification of severe combined immunodeficiency by T-cell receptor excision circles quantification using neonatal Guthrie cards. J Pediatr 2009;155(6):829–33.

19. Douek DC, McFarland RD, Keiser PH, et al. Changes in thymic function with age and during the treatment of HIV infection. Nature 1998;396(6712):690–5.

20. Verschuren MC, Wolvers-Tettero IL, Breit TM, et al. Preferential rearrangements of the T cell receptor-delta-deleting elements in human T cells. J Immunol 1997;158: 1208–16.

21. Chan K, Puck JM. Development of population-based newborn screening for severe combined immunodeficiency. J Allergy Clin Immunol 2005;115(2):391–8.

22. Hazenberg MD, Otto SA, Cohen Stuart JW, et al. Increased cell division but not thymic dysfunction rapidly affects the T-cell receptor excision circle content of the naive T cell population in HIV-1 infection. Nat Med 2000;6(9):1036–42.

23. Routes J, Verbsky J. Newborn screening for severe combined immunodeficiency. Curr Allergy Asthma Rep 2018;18(34):1–7.

24. Shearer WT, Dunn E, Notarangelo LD, et al. Establishing diagnostic criteria for severe combined immunodeficiency disease (SCID), leaky SCID, and Omenn syndrome: the Primary Immune Deficiency Treatment Consortium experience. J Allergy Clin Immunol 2014;133(4):1092–8.

25. Villa A, Notarangelo LD, Roifman CM. Omenn syndrome: inflammation in leaky severe combined immunodeficiency. J Allergy Clin Immunol 2008;122(6):1082–6.

26. Jyonouchi S, Jongco AM, Puck J, et al. Immunodeficiencies associated with abnormal newborn screening for T cell and B cell lymphopenia. J Clin Immunol 2017;37:363–74.

27. Mauracher AA, Pagliarulo F, Faes L, et al. Causes of low neonatal T-cell receptor excision circles: a systematic review. J Allergy Clin Immunol Pract 2017;5: 1457–60.e22.

28. Grazioli S, Bennett M, Hildebrand KJ, et al. Limitation of TREC-based newborn screening for ZAP70 severe combined immunodeficiency. Clin Immunol 2014; 153:209.

29. Kuo CY, Chase J, Garcia Lloret M, et al. Newborn screening for severe combined immunodeficiency does not identify bare lymphocyte syndrome. J Allergy Clin Immunol 2013;131:1693.

30. Kwan A, Abraham RS, Currier R, et al. Newborn screening for severe combined immunodeficiency in 11 screening programs in the United States. JAMA 2014; 312:729–38.

31. Verbsky J, Thakar M, Routes J. The Wisconsin approach to newborn screening for severe combined immunodeficiency. J Allergy Clin Immunol 2012;129(3): 622–7.

32. van der Spek J, Groenwold RH, van der Burg M, et al. TREC based newborn screening for severe combined immunodeficiency disease: a systematic review. J Clin Immunol 2015;35(4):416–30.

33. Dorsey MJ, Dvorak CC, Cowan MJ, et al. Treatment of infants identified as having severe combined immunodeficiency by means of newborn screening. J Allergy Clin Immunol 2017;139(3):733–42.

34. Vogel BH, Bonagura V, Weinberg GA, et al. Newborn screening for SCID in New York State: experience from the first two years. J Clin Immunol 2014;34(3): 289–303.

35. Kwan A, Church JA, Cowan MJ, et al. Newborn screening for severe combined immunodeficiency and T-cell lymphopenia in California: results of the first 2 years. J Allergy Clin Immunol 2013;132(1):140–50.

36. Immunocompromised children. In: Pickering LK, Baker CJ, Kimberlin DW, et al, editors. The red book: 2009 report to the committee on infections diseases.

28th edition. Elk Grove Village (IL): American Academy of Pediatrics; 2009. p. 72–86.

37. Griffith LM, Cowan MJ, Notarangelo LD, et al. Improving cellular therapy for primary immune deficiency diseases: recognition, diagnosis, and management. J Allergy Clin Immunol 2009;124:1152–60.e12.

38. Thakar MS, Hintermeyer MK, Gries MG, et al. A practical approach to newborn screening for severe combined immunodeficiency using the T cell receptor excision circle assay. Front Immunol 2017;8:1470.

39. Yu H, Zhang VW, Stray-Pedersen A, et al. Rapid molecular diagnostics of severe primary immunodeficiency determined by using targeted next-generation sequencing. J Allergy Clin Immunol 2016;138:1142–451.e2.

40. Cowan MJ, Gennery AR. Radiation-sensitive severe combined immunodeficiency: the arguments for and against conditioning before hematopoietic cell transplantation–what to do? J Allergy Clin Immunol 2015;136(5):1178–85.

41. Pai SY, Logan BR, Griffith LM, et al. Transplantation outcomes for severe combined immunodeficiency, 2000–2009. N Engl J Med 2014;371:434–46.

42. Heimall J, Logan BR, Cowan MJ, et al. Immune reconstitution and survival of 100 SCID patients post-hematopoietic cell transplant: a PIDTC natural history study. Blood 2017;130:2718–27.

New Treatments for Asthma

Jenny Huang, MD[a], Milind Pansare, MD[b],*

KEYWORDS

- Severe asthma • Asthma endotypes • Biologics
- Long-acting antimuscarinic agents • Bronchial thermoplasty

KEY POINTS

- Asthma is a complex, heterogeneous chronic airway disease with high prevalence of uncontrolled disease.
- New therapies, including biologics, are now available to treat T2 high asthma.
- Treatment of T2 low asthma remains a challenge.
- Asthma guidelines need be to updated to incorporate new therapeutics.

INTRODUCTION

Asthma was reported as the most prevalent chronic respiratory disease worldwide and had twice as many prevalent cases as chronic obstructive pulmonary disease.[1] Globally, the prevalence of asthma increased by 13% to more than 358 million persons from 1990 to 2015.[1] In the United States, the prevalence of asthma was estimated at 26 million persons in 2010, with 19 million adults (>18 years) and more than 7 million children (<17 years).[2] The total annual costs (including medical care, indirect) for medically treated asthma is estimated at $82 billion.[3] Unfortunately, uncontrolled asthma is common and associated with increased costs, increased health care use, and decreased economic productivity.[4]

To improve care of patients with asthma, in 1991, National Asthma Education and Prevention Program (NAEPP) produced the first expert panel report (EPR) on guidelines for the diagnosis and management of asthma with comprehensive updates. The last guidelines were published in 2007 as EPR-3 report. EPR-3 is a comprehensive scientific evidence-based guideline for delivering best care for adults and children with asthma. It defined goals of asthma treatment as "asthma control" based on 2 domains: reduce current impairment, defined as "frequency and intensity of symptoms

[a] Division of Allergy and Immunology, Department of Pediatrics, Children's Hospital of Michigan, Suite #4022, 4th Floor, 3950 Beaubien Boulevard, Detroit, MI 48201, USA; [b] Division of Allergy and Immunology, Department of Pediatrics, Children's Hospital of Michigan, Pediatric Specialty Center, Wayne State University, Suite # 4018, 4th Floor, 3950 Beaubien Boulevard, Detroit, MI 48201, USA
* Corresponding author.
E-mail address: mpansare@dmc.org

Pediatr Clin N Am 66 (2019) 925–939
https://doi.org/10.1016/j.pcl.2019.06.001
0031-3955/19/© 2019 Elsevier Inc. All rights reserved.

and functional limitations," and reduce risks, defined as "likelihood of exacerbations, decline of lung functions, and side effects of medications." The recommended 6-step EPR-3–guided traditional drug treatment is effective in attaining treatment goals in most mild to moderate severe asthma. However, despite use of effective drug therapies, asthma control is suboptimal in most patients with moderate to severe chronic asthma.[4] The outcome of uncontrolled asthma is significant health care use, risks for airway intubation in both adults and children,[4] and a high risk of death.[5] Many promising newer agents and biologics likely to improve asthma outcomes are now available to treat primarily T2 asthma, which is reviewed here.

WHO ARE THE CANDIDATES FOR EMERGING THERAPIES?

Candidates for emerging therapies are patients with severe refractory asthma. Identification of uncontrolled or severe asthma is an essential first step in asthma management. Severe refractory asthma per the European Respiratory Society/American Thoracic Society guidelines[6] is defined as a patient with refractory asthma in whom alternate diagnosis is excluded, comorbidities treated, triggers removed, compliance checked but remains poorly controlled or with frequent, severe exacerbations despite prescription of high-intensity treatment (NAEPP-EPR-3, step 5 or 6) or who require systemic corticosteroids to maintain control. Patients in whom poor control is due to nonadherence, untreated comorbid conditions, or poor inhaler technique can be categorized as "difficult-to-treat" severe asthma and are likely to improve with high-dose or add-on traditional therapy and by addressing the interfering factors.[6] Some of the factors to be considered before considering targeted therapies are listed in **Table 1**.

AIRWAY INFLAMMATORY PHENOTYPES

Recent studies have increasingly characterized severe asthma into 2 inflammatory subtypes: a type 2 high, with high levels of eosinophils, and a type 2 low, or non-T2, with low levels of eosinophil endotypes with each having distinct physiologic and clinical characteristics.[7,8] Analysis of sputum samples from the patients in the Belgian Severe Asthma Registry showed that approximately half (55%) of severe asthma cases were eosinophilic, with the remainder having other inflammatory phenotypes, including neutrophilic (21%), paucigranulocytic (18%), and mixed granulocytic (6%).[9] These investigators also presented criteria defining type 2 high and type 2 low phenotypes, with the type 2 high phenotype being defined as a sputum eosinophil count greater than 3% or the presence of both exhaled nitric oxide greater than 27 ppb and blood eosinophil count greater than 188/μmL.[8] The 2 primary endotypes: T2 high and T2 low, are based on activity of T2 helper (Th2) cells and type 2 innate lymphoid cell activity (ILC2).[7,8] The T2 high is characterized by eosinophilic inflammation and elevated type 2 cytokines, such as interleukins -4 IL-4, IL-5, IL-13 produced by the Th2 and ILC2 cells and regulated by transcription factor GATA-3. Epithelial factors like IL-25, IL-33, and thymic stromal lymphopoietin (TSLP) also regulate expression of this T2 cytokines.[8,10] IL-4 action results in the production of immunoglobulin E (IgE) and subsequent activation of mast cells (ckit-SCF) and activation and recruitment of eosinophils through IL-5 cytokine. IL-13 acts on smooth muscles to induce hyperresponsiveness and remodeling. Mast cells also synthesize prostaglandin D_2 (PGD$_2$), which stimulates upstream cells, and basophils, eosinophils through its actions at the receptor known as chemoattractant receptor-homologous molecules (CRTH2) expressed on Th2 cells. Mast cells produce multiple mediators and cytokines that cause airway smooth-muscle contraction, eosinophil infiltration, remodeling, and

Table 1
Evaluations before considering targeted therapies

1. Confirm asthma diagnosis	Assess symptoms, airflow limitations, and if necessary, airway hyperresponsiveness Periodic lung functions Exclude other diagnosis (eg, vocal cord dysfunction, ABPA, AERD [aspirin-exacerbated respiratory airway disease]) Consider specialist referral
2. Adequate trial of medications	EPR-3–guided step-based therapy, high-dose inhaled steroids plus LABA Add-on treatments: LTRA, theophylline, oral steroids Immunotherapy Antimuscarinic agents: Tiotropium Adherence Pharmacy refills
3. Optimize inhaled treatment	Patient education, inhaler techniques Adherence Written asthma action plans Multidisciplinary team approach Asthma control measurement
4. Comorbid diseases	Allergic rhinitis Sinusitis Gastroesophageal reflux disease Mental health Obesity Social issues: Insurance coverage, access to health care Emotional stress
5. Environmental triggers	Allergen control (eg, dust mites, pet dander, mold, rodents, cockroaches) Cigarette smoking

Abbreviations: ABPA, allergic bronchopulmonary aspergillosis; AERD, aspirin exacerbated respiratory disease; LABA, long acting beta agonist; LTRA, leukotriene receptor antagonist.

amplification of the inflammatory cascade through additional cytokine production, IL-3, IL-4, IL-5, and IL-9. Many of these cytokines, IL-4/IL-13, IL-5, and mediators like IgE are targets of biologic therapies.[10] T2 asthma is likely to be associated with biomarkers like elevated eosinophils (blood, sputum), fractional exhaled nitric oxide (FeNO), serum periostin, and dipeptidyl peptidase-4.[7,8] Subjects with T2 asthma are likely to be responsive to corticosteroid treatments but with variable outcomes and also responsive to the newer biologics.[11,12]

T2 Low Asthma

The pathophysiology of T2 low asthma is not well understood but is characterized by the absence of T2 markers of activation and eosinophilia. Instead, T2 low asthma is marked by neutrophilic or paucigranulocytic inflammation as a result of the activation of Th1 and/or Th17 cells and the release of their specific cytokines, such as interferon-γ (IFN-y) and IL-17.[8,11,12] In addition, T2 low inflammation may be driven by the release of other proinflammatory cytokines, such as tumor necrosis factor-α (TNF-α), IL-1b, IL-6, IL-8, and the IL-12 family.[8,11,12] Subjects with T2 low asthma usually have a later disease onset, have a lack a history of environmental allergies, and are less responsive to corticosteroids[12] (**Table 2**).

Some of the targeted agents studied for treating T2 high/T2 low asthma are listed in **Table 3**.

Table 2
Asthma endotypes[11,12]

Endotypes	T2 High Asthma	T2 Low Asthma
Predominant cell in airways or sputum	Eosinophils	Neutrophils or paucigranulocyte
Predominant cells and cytokines involved		
Epithelium	TSLP, IL-33	IL-8, IL-23
Neutrophils		Proteases, ROS
Eosinophils/mast cells	IL-4, IL-5, IL-9, CRTH2/PGD2	
Th1		IFN-γ, IL-17, IL-22
Th2	IL-4, IL-5, IL-9, L-13, CRTH2/PGD2	
Th17		IL-17, 1L-22, 1L-23, CXCR2
ILC	ILC2-IL-4, IL-5, IL-13, IL-9, Areg	ILC1 & 3, IL-17, IL-22
FeNO	>27 ppb	
Eosinophils: Sputum Peripheral blood eosinophils	>2% in sputum >150 cells/μL	
Therapies	Anticytokines, anti-IgE	

Abbreviation: ROS, reactive oxygen species.

Table 3
T2 high/T2 low asthma treatment agents

T2 High Agents		Possible T2 Low Treatment Agents	
Anti-IgE	Omalizumab, ligelizumab (QGE031) Quilizumab (RG7449)	Airway smooth muscle	Bronchial thermoplasty[a]
IL-5	Mepolizumab Reslizumab	Neutrophils Anti-CXCR2 Anti–granulocyte-macrophage colony-stimulating factor (GM CSF)	Macrolides
IL-5Rα	Benralizumab	TNF-α	Adalimumab, Etarnecept
IL-13Rβ	Lebrikizumab	Th17 pathway	Secukinumab, Brodalumab
IL-13	Tralokinumab		
IL-4α	Dupilumab		
GATA3	GATA3 DNAzyme		
TSLP	Tezepelumab		
PDG2-antagonist	Fevipiprant		
ILC2	Anti-CRTH2		

Abbreviation: CXCR2, CXC chemokine receptor 2; IL, interleukins; TNF, tumor necrosis factor; TSLP, thymic stromal lymphopoietin.
[a] Bronchial thermoplasty likely to be effective for both T2 high and T2 low endotype.

Anti–Immunoglobulin E

Omalizumab is a recombinant, humanized murine monoclonal IgG1 anti-IgE antibody that binds to the Fc region of IgE, preventing IgE from binding to cell-surface receptors of mast cells and basophils and thus inhibiting the release of inflammatory mediators that can cause allergic inflammation and asthma exacerbation.[13] Omalizumab was first approved in 2002 for treating individuals 12 years and older and later in 2016 for patients aged 6 to 12 years with moderate or severe uncontrolled allergic asthma treated with inhaled corticosteroids and perennial allergen sensitivity.[14] A meta-analysis of 3429 patients aged 5 to 79 years from 8 double-blind, placebo-controlled trials showed that omalizumab reduced the exacerbation rate as well as the ICS dose and rescue medication use.[15] Other studies have also demonstrated improved quality of life,[14] meaningful improvement in lung functions (improved forced expiratory volume in 1 second [FEV1]),[16] prevention of exacerbation of fall season asthma in inner-city children (6–17 years) with severe asthma (PROSE study),[17] and effectiveness in nonallergic asthma.[18] Pooled data from randomized trials indicate that adverse events (AEs) in patients who received omalizumab are similar to those in patients who received control drugs or placebo.[19] The most common AEs were nasopharyngitis, headache, respiratory tract infection, and sinusitis.[19] Omalizumab has a boxed warning for anaphylaxis and a safety warning for malignancy.[14] Hypersensitivity reactions occurred rarely, with anaphylaxis occurring in 0.14% of patients receiving omalizumab compared with 0.07% in patients in control groups.[19] In clinical trials, malignant neoplasms were observed in 0.5% of patients treated with omalizumab (vs 0.18% of patients who received placebo). In a pooled analysis[20] of clinical data and a prospective postmarketing safety study (The Epidemiologic Study of Xolair) found that omalizumab was not associated with an increased risk of malignancy.[21]

How Long to Treat?

Omalizumab is administered subcutaneously (SQ) 75 mg to 375 mg every 2 to 4 weeks; exact dose is determined by patient's serum IgE and body weight.[14] Patients who failed to show improvement should be reexamined at 16 to 24 weeks of therapy for possible continuation of omalizumab.[22] The optimal duration of therapy is not well understood, but prolonged treatment without interruption is desirable as loss of asthma control is known, particularly in patients with eosinophilia, elevated periostin, and FeNO.[22,23] Studies suggest sustained improved clinical improvement[23] and cost-effectiveness with long-term treatments.[24]

Ligelizumab, another anti-IgE monoclonal antibody, has 30 to 50 times greater affinity for IgE than omalizumab. An open-label, multicenter, extension study was designed to evaluate the long-term safety of SQ 240 mg QGE031 (ligelizumab) given every 4 weeks for 52 weeks in allergic asthma patients (clinicaltrials.gov; #NCT02075008) who had completed the initial study (CQGE031B2201). The study was prematurely terminated after core study CQGE031B2201 failed to meet the primary objective of demonstrating superiority for QGE031 versus placebo.

Anti–Interleukin-5 Treatment

Three biologics targeting IL-5, either blocking IL-5 (mepolizumab, reslizumab) or IL-5 receptor (benralizumab), have been shown to reduce blood eosinophils and clinical improvement of asthma. However, a head-to-head efficacy comparison study to date is lacking.

Table 4
Mepolizumab studies

Clinical Studies	Outcome	
DREAM (Dose Ranging, Efficacy, and Safety with Mepolizumab in Severe Asthma) study[26] • Randomized, double-blind, placebo-controlled trial • Adults and >12 y • History of recurrent severe asthma exacerbations and eosinophilic inflammation	Mepolizumab was found to reduce • Blood and sputum eosinophils • Rate of exacerbations per patient per year • Number of exacerbations requiring hospitalization or ED visit • In addition, it delayed the time to first exacerbation	No significant difference in • FEV1 • Asthma quality-of-life questionnaire scores, or Asthma Control Questionnaire (ACQ) scores No pediatric patients were actually enrolled in this study even though eligibility included 12 y and older
MENSA (Mepolizumab as Adjunctive Therapy in Patients with Severe Asthma) trial[27] • A double-blind, double-dummy, and 32-wk study • Patients 12–82 y old with recurrent asthma exacerbations and eosinophilic inflammation despite high-dose ICS	Mepolizumab was found to improve • FEV • St. George's Respiratory Questionnaire (SGRQ; assesses quality of life) scores • Rates of all exacerbations (reduced by approximately 50%), and • Exacerbations requiring a hospitalization or ED visit reduced by 32%–61%.	Improvement in ACQ scores did not meet criteria for clinical importance
SIRIUS (Oral Glucocorticoid-Sparing Effect of Mepolizumab in Eosinophilic Asthma) study[28] • A randomized, double-blind trial • Patients >12 y old with serum eosinophilia and who required maintenance OCS for at least 6 mo	Mepolizumab was found to allow reduction in OCS dose compared with placebo Mepolizumab-treated group • Had a 50% median reduction in daily OCS use from baseline • Had a reduction in annualized rate of asthma exacerbations by 32% • Improved ACQ scores despite reducing their OCS dose	There was not a significant improvement in FEV1 by the end of the 24-wk trial

Abbreviation: OCS, oral corticosteroids.
Data from Refs.[26–28]

1. Mepolizumab

Mepolizumab is a recombinant immunoglobulin G1 IgG1k (Ig1Gk) anti–IL-5 antibody, first approved in 2015, for treatment of severe eosinophilic asthma based on clinical studies.[25]

Mepolizumab studies for eosinophilic asthma thus show reduced exacerbations, emergency room visits, and hospitalization[26,27] and improved asthma quality-of-life scores and FEV1 and oral corticosteroid-sparing effects.[28] It is also approved for eosinophilic granulomatosis with polyangiitis treatment while explored for potential benefit for eosinophilic esophagitis.[29,30]

Table 5
Mepolizumab: summary

Pros	Cons
Available as 100-mg lyophilized powder to reconstitute before use	Expensive

Recommended dose[a]: FDA approved
Adult and children >12 y:
  100 mg SQ every 4 wk
Children 6–11 y: 40 mg SQ every 4 wk
Indication:
  Add-on treatment of severe
    eosinophilic asthma >12 y of age
  Screening: Eosinophil
    count of >150 cells/μL or >300
    cells/μL within past 12 mo
	Safety warning: Hypersensitivity reactions-rare.
	  Herpes zoster infection,
	  vaccinate before starting therapy
	Helminth infections: Treat before
	  initiating treatment
	Common adverse reaction: Headache,
	  fatigue, local injection site reactions,
	  pruritus, eczema, abdominal pain, muscle spasm

Other potential uses-not FDA approved
  Eosinophilic granulomatosis
    with polyangiitis[29]
  Eosinophilic esophagitis?[30]
	No data of use during pregnancy
	  and lactation

[a] Nucala (mepolizumab) Package Insert. 2017.[25]

2. Reslizumab is a humanized monoclonal antibody (IG4) against IL-5 blocking binding of IL-5 to IL-5 receptors.

Clinical studies[31,32] showed reslizumab decreases asthma exacerbation rates, improves FEV1, and improves asthma quality-of-life scores. As with mepolizumab, greater clinical benefit is noted in patients with higher blood eosinophil levels (>400 cells/μL).

3. Benralizumab

Benralizumab is a humanized monoclonal antibody that targets the IL-5 receptor α subunit of eosinophils and basophils, causing rapid, direct, and near depletion of eosinophils by antibody-dependent cytotoxicity. It is shown to decrease eosinophils in airways, sputum, bone marrow, and blood.

Benralizumab was Food and Drug Administration (FDA) approved in November 2017 for add-on maintenance treatment of patients aged 12 years and older with severe asthma, with eosinophilic phenotype asthma. It has been shown to have corticosteroid-sparing effects and improved FEV1 and also decreased exacerbation rates (overall 40% at 12 weeks, $P = .01$) following a single dose administered in the emergency department (ED).[36]

A Cochrane systematic review evaluated 13 studies that involved 6000 participants with severe eosinophilic asthma treated with anti–IL-5 therapy: 4 used mepolizumab, 4 used reslizumab, and 5 used benralizumab. All the anti–IL-5 treatments assessed reduced rates of clinically significant asthma exacerbations by approximately 50%. It also showed a small but statistically significant improvement in mean pr-bronchodilator FEV1 of 0.08 to 0.11 L. The investigators concluded that further research is needed on finding biomarkers for assessing treatment response, optimal duration, and long-term effects of such treatment, risk of relapse on withdrawal, on effects in patients without eosinophilia, and in younger children (<12 years), and also comparing different anti–IL-5 treatments with each other (**Tables 4–9**).[37]

Table 6
Reslizumab clinical asthma studies and outcomes

Reslizumab Clinical Asthma Studies	Outcomes	Comment
Two phase 3 trials[31] 52-wk, duplicate, multicenter, double-blind, parallel-group, randomized, placebo-controlled • Patients aged 12–75 y with inadequately controlled asthma on medium- to high-dose ICS and • Blood eosinophil count ≥ 400	Reslizumab showed • Decreased annual rate of exacerbations by 50%–59% compared with placebo • Reducing eosinophil counts in both blood and sputum • Improvement in time to first exacerbation, FEV1, asthma control scores, and quality-of-life scores	Suggests eosinophil count >400 cells/µL is important surrogate marker for response to therapy
16-wk, randomized, double-blind, placebo-controlled, phase 3 trial[32] • Patients ≥ 18 y old • Eosinophil count: Broad range	Improved outcomes	Reslizumab did not result in clinically meaningful effects on lung function and symptom control in patients with baseline eosinophils < 400 cells/µL

ANTI–INTERLEUKIN-4/INTERLEUKIN-13

Dupilumab is a humanized monoclonal antibody that binds to the IL-4Rα subunit, which inhibits both IL-4 and IL-13 signaling and decreases IgE production by approximately 40%.[38] Recent studies[39,40] show dupilumab treatment (100-300 mg) for severe asthma results in decreased exacerbations and improved control of asthma symptoms with concomitant reduction of T2 biomarkers, and with effects independent of blood eosinophil count. The increase in eosinophil count with treatment is likely due to blockage of migration into the tissues rather than overproduction.

Dupilumab is approved for treatment of moderate-severe atopic dermatitis in adults. It is under FDA review as an add-on maintenance treatment of moderate to severe eosinophilic asthma for patients 12 years of age and older (**Table 10**).

Anti–Interleukin-13

Cytokine IL-13 plays important role in asthma remodeling and inflammation. Three humanized monoclonal IL-13 antibodies have been studied for the treatment of asthma:

Table 7
Reslizumab summary

Use	Caution
FDA approved for those >18 y Available as 100 mg/10 mL single-use vial • Infusion given over 20–50 min • Intravenous use • Dose: 3 mg/kg given every 4 wk • More effective with eosinophil count >400 cells/µL	Intravenous use ONLY and needs to be administered in supervised facility Not approved for any other eosinophilic conditions
SQ preparation under development	Adverse events (AE): Worsening of asthma, upper respiratory tract infection (URTI), headache, and oropharyngeal pain FDA warning for anaphylaxis

Table 8
Benralizumab clinical studies and outcomes

Benralizumab Clinical Studies	Outcomes	Comment
The SIROCCO study, phase 3[33] • 48-wk, randomized, multicenter, placebo-controlled • 1204 patients aged 12–75 y old including 53 patients between 12 and 17 y old • Physician-diagnosed asthma for at least 1 y and at least 2 exacerbations while on high-dose ICS plus LABA in the previous year	Benralizumab reduced • Annual asthma exacerbation rates • Improved lung function when dosed every 4 or 8 wk	
The CALIMA phase 3 trial[34] • 56-wk, randomized, multicenter, double-blind, placebo-controlled, and • Patients 12–75 y old, 1306 patients, including 55 patients between 12 and 17 y old • Severe asthma uncontrolled with medium- to high-dose ICS plus LABA and at least 2 exacerbations in the previous year	Supported the SIROCCO findings Significantly lowered exacerbation rates and improved FEV1 in the benralizumab group Improvement in FEV1 was evident as early as 4 wk and sustained throughout the study	FEV1 is an important clinical parameter when assessing patient response to benralizumab
ZONDA trial • A 28-wk, randomized, double-blind, parallel-group and placebo-controlled trial • Only 18 y or older • Uncontrolled asthma with high-dose inhaled steroid plus LABA • Investigated the oral corticosteroid-sparing effect with placebo[35]	Benralizumab allowed decreased use of maintenance OCS, with the median final oral steroid dose decreased by 75% with benralizumab vs by 25% placebo	

anrukinzumab, lebrikizumab, and tralokinumab. Lebrikizumab[41] and tralokinumab[42] have failed to show any promising and consistent results favoring further trial in the treatment of asthma.

Antithymic Stromal Lymphopoietin and Anti–Interleukin-33

Two novel targets, TSLP and IL-33, for biologic therapy are being investigated. TSLP is an upstream cytokine potentiating T2 immune response through multiple mechanisms and thus potential for broader downstream effects. Tezepelumab is an investigational

Table 9 Benralizumab summary	
Use	**Caution**
FDA approved in 2017 for more than 12 year of age	Patients with eosinophil counts <300 cells/ μL may have a smaller benefits
Available as 30 mg/mL in single-dose prefilled syringe	Not approved for other eosinophilic conditions
Recommended dose: Fixed 30-mg SQ dose, with first 3 doses given every 4 wk and the subsequent doses every 8 wk	AEs: Headache, pharyngitis, local reactions Cost
Single dose for acute asthma exacerbation[36] Oral corticosteroid sparing? Improved FEV1	

human IgG2 monoclonal antibody binding to TSLP, preventing its binding to TSLP receptor and thus its effects. Two phase 3 studies are assessing efficacy of tezelepumab on annual rate of asthma exacerbations (NAVIGATOR),[43] and another is evaluating percent reduction from baseline oral corticosteroids dose (SOURCE)[44] in patients aged 18 to 80 years.

Table 10 Dupilumab clinical trials and outcomes		
Dupilumab Clinical Trials	**Outcome**	**Comment**
The Liberty Asthma QUEST phase 3 trial[39] • 52-wk, randomized, double-blind, placebo-controlled, parallel group • Aged >12 y and older • 1902 patients (107 were adolescents) were uncontrolled asthmatics • Dose 200 mg, and 300 mg every 2 wk	Dupilumab • 47.7% reduction of exacerbations in the overall group, with 65.8% reduction in those with baseline eosinophil counts of ≥ 300 cells/μL • FEV1 at 12 wk, increased by 0.32 L	Similar results with higher 300-mg dose of dupilumab • Greater treatment effects with increasing baseline levels of blood eosinophils and FeNO
Liberty Asthma Venture Trial assessed the OCS-sparing effect of dupilumab[40] • 24-wk, randomized, double-blind, placebo-controlled, and phase 3 trial • Patients ≥ 12 y old with severe OCS-dependent asthma regardless of eosinophil levels	Dupilumab, treatment • 70.1% reduction in OCS dose compared with 41.9% with placebo • At 24 wk, despite the reduction in OCS dose, patients on dupilumab still had 59% fewer exacerbations in the overall population and 71% fewer exacerbations in those with eosinophil counts ≥ 300 cells/μL • At 24 wk, dupilumab improved lung function; FEV_1 improved by 0.22 L (15%) in the overall population and by 0.32 L (25%) in those with eosinophil counts ≥ 300 cells/μL	Benefits were more pronounced in patients with a higher baseline blood eosinophil count and FeNO level AEs: Injection site reactions, URTI, headache Increased blood eosinophil counts

PGD2 is a prostanoid produced mostly by the mast cells in allergic diseases. Prostanoid receptors and the homologous receptor mutant molecule expressed on Th2 (CRTH2) cells have been shown to be the major PGD2-related receptors that have central roles in the regulation of the functions of several cells crucial in allergic diseases.[45] Fevipiprant (QAW039) is administered orally and is an antagonist of PGD2 receptor CRTH2, thus inhibiting the migration and activation of eosinophils, basophils, and T lymphocytes into the airway tissues and blocking the PGD2-driven release of Th2 cytokines.[46] Preliminary data confirm a good safety profile and improvement of FEV1, especially in patients with more severe obstruction.[47] In a subsequent randomized, single-center, double-blind, parallel group, placebo-controlled study on 61 patients with moderate to severe asthma, fevipiprant reduced eosinophilic airways and sputum inflammation and was well tolerated.[48]

T2 Low Asthma

T2 low asthma is marked by neutrophilic or pauci-granulocytic inflammation as a result of activation of Th1 and/or Th17 cells and release of cytokines, such as IFN-γ and IL-17, TNF-α, IL-1β, IL-6, IL-8, and IL-12 family.[11,12] T2 low asthma is characterized by later onset of asthma, lack of environmental allergies, and less responsiveness to corticosteroids. Several clinical trials assessing monoclonal antibodies against TNF-α (adalimumab),[49] TNF-receptor-IgG1 fusion protein (Etanercept),[50] and Th17A (Secukinumab)[51] or IL-17 receptor (brodalumab)[52] have failed to show consistent meaningful or statistically significant benefits. Macrolide antibiotics have been shown to improve neutrophilia-associated markers and quality of life, but not lung function or asthma control in subjects with moderate to severe T2 low asthma.[53] T2 low asthma thus is poorly understood at this time, and perhaps the chosen targets are not key elements in the pathophysiology of T2 low asthma.

Bronchial Thermoplasty

In 2010, the FDA had approved the Alair Bronchial Thermoplasty System (Boston Scientific, Marlborough, MA, USA) for the treatment of severe persistent asthma in patients 18 years and older whose asthma is not well controlled with inhaled corticosteroids and long-acting beta-agonists (LABAs). Bronchial thermoplasty (BT) is an endoscopic procedure that targets airway remodeling by delivering temperature-controlled radiofrequency energy to the airway wall by a disposable catheter introduced into the bronchoscope operating channel (Alair).[54] BT is a one-time procedure that is completed after 3 treatments performed 20 days apart. It reduces excess airway smooth muscle and inflammation associated with asthma and thereby improved control.[54] Several studies have demonstrated improved asthma symptoms, quality of life,[54,55] reduced exacerbations, and also long-term safety and effectiveness in terms of reducing serious exacerbations.[56]

BT may be considered in patients older than 18 years with severe asthma and FEV1 $\geq$60% of the predicted values and unsuitable for the currently available biologics (omalizumab or mepolizumab), in patients with frequent exacerbations and hospitalization, regardless of T2 high or T2 low asthma endotypes.[54,55] Current limitations include access to experienced specialist and institute offering BT, cost and insurance coverage, proper selection of patient, and both short- and long-term risks and benefits.

Long-Acting Muscarinic Antagonists

Inhibition of muscarinic receptors of the bronchioles causes relaxation of smooth muscle and also is shown to reduce inflammation and asthma-related airway remodeling in preclinical asthma models.[57] Tiotropium is the first long-acting muscarinic antagonist approved for use in asthma in 2014. It was also licensed for use as a once-daily maintenance add-on therapy in patients aged 6 years and older in the United States in early 2017. The Global Initiative for Asthma 2018 recommends tiotropium for severe asthma as step 4 treatment before using oral steroids or biologics. Tiotropium appears to be efficacious independent of asthma phenotypes[58] and shown to be cost-effective, reducing the needs for expensive biologics.[59]

SUMMARY

Asthma is a chronic heterogeneous and complex airway inflammatory disease with varied response to therapy. In the pursuit of achieving control in severe asthma, improved knowledge of chronic airway inflammatory pathways has resulted in the development of new targeted therapies mostly to treat a T2 high asthma. Some of the drugs have received FDA approval owing to safety and significant clinical benefits demonstrated in clinical trials. Choosing these agents is a formidable task because there is lack of clear identifiable "treatable traits" or "ideal biomarkers" to guide such therapies. New guidance to choosing the "ideal" patient and incorporating multimodal treatments for best and cost-effective use of biologics, newer agents, and non-pharmacologic treatments like BT needs to be updated in the guidelines for asthma treatment in the immediate future.

REFERENCES

1. Chronic Respiratory Disease Collaborators. Global, regional, and national deaths, prevalence, disability-adjusted life years, and years lived with disability for chronic obstructive pulmonary disease and asthma, 1990-2015: a systematic analysis for the Global Burden of Disease Study 2015. Lancet Respir Med 2017;5: 691–706.
2. Akinbami LJ, Moorman JE, Bailey C, et al. Trends in asthma prevalence, health care use, and mortality in the United States, 2001-2010. NCHS Data Brief 2012;(94):1–8.
3. Nurmagambetov T, Kuwahara R, Garbe P. The economic burden of asthma in the United States, 2008-2013. Ann Am Thorac Soc 2018;15:348–56.
4. Sullivan PW, Slejko JF, Ghushchyan VH, et al. The relationship between asthma, asthma control and economic outcomes in the United States. J Asthma 2014;51: 769–78.
5. Omachi TA, Iribarren C, Sarkar U, et al. Risk factors for death in adults with severe asthma. Ann Allergy Asthma Immunol 2008;101:130–6.
6. Chung KF, Wenzel SE, Brozek JL, et al. International ERS/ATS guidelines on definition, evaluation and treatment of severe asthma. Eur Respir J 2014;43:34–73.
7. Wenzel SE. Asthma phenotypes: the evolution from clinical to molecular approaches. Nat Med 2012;18:716–25.
8. Wenzel SE, Schwartz LB, Langmack EL, et al. Evidence that severe asthma can be divided pathologically into two inflammatory subtypes with distinct physiologic and clinical characteristics. Am J Respir Crit Care Med 1999;160:1001–8.
9. Schleich F, Brusselle G, Louis R, et al. Heterogeneity of phenotypes in severe asthmatics. The Belgian Severe Asthma Registry (BSAR). Respir Med 2014; 108:1723–32.
10. Lambrecht BN, Hammad H. The immunology of asthma. Nat Immunol 2015;16: 45–56.

11. Muraro A, Lemanske RF Jr, Hellings PW, et al. Precision medicine in patients with allergic diseases: airway diseases and atopic dermatitis—PRACTALL document of the European Academy of Allergy and Clinical Immunology and the American Academy of Allergy, Asthma & Immunology. J Allergy Clin Immunol 2016;137: 1347–58.

12. Stokes JR, Casale TB. Characterization of asthma endotypes: implications for therapy. Ann Allergy Asthma Immunol 2016;117:121–5.

13. Strunk RC, Bloomberg GR. Omalizumab for asthma. N Engl J Med 2006;354: 2689–95.

14. Xolair [prescribing information]. South San Francisco, Calif: Genentech/Novartis. 2016. Available at. http://www.gene.com/download/pdf/xolair prescribing.pdf. Accessed July 28, 2016.

15. Rodrigo GJ, Neffen H, Castro-Rodriguez JA. Efficacy and safety of subcutaneous omalizumab vs placebo as add-on therapy to corticosteroids for children and adults with asthma: a systematic review. Chest 2011;139:28–35.

16. Humbert M, Busse W, Hanania NA, et al. Omalizumab in asthma: an update on recent developments. J Allergy Clin Immunol Pract 2014;2:525–36.e1.

17. Teach SJ, Gill MA, Togias A, et al. Preseasonal treatment with either omalizumab or an inhaled corticosteroid boost to prevent fall asthma exacerbations. J Allergy Clin Immunol 2015;136(6):1476–85.

18. Menzella F, Piro R, Facciolongo N, et al. Long-term benefits of omalizumab in a patient with severe non-allergic asthma. Allergy Asthma Clin Immunol 2011; 7(1):9.

19. Corren J, Casale TB, Lanier B, et al. Safety and tolerability of omalizumab. Clin Exp Allergy 2009;39:788–97.

20. Busse W, Buhl R, Fernandez Vidaurre C, et al. Omalizumab and the risk of malignancy: results from a pooled analysis. J Allergy Clin Immunol 2012;129:983–9.e6.

21. Long A, Rahmaoui A, Rothman KJ, et al. Incidence of malignancy in patients with moderate-to-severe asthma treated with or without omalizumab. J Allergy Clin Immunol 2014;134:560–7.e4.

22. Hanania NA, Wenzel S, Rosén K, et al. Exploring the effects of omalizumab in allergic asthma: an analysis of biomarkers in the EXTRA study. Am J Respir Crit Care Med 2013;187(8):804–11.

23. Ledford D, Busse W, Trzaskoma B, et al. A randomized multicenter study evaluating Xolair persistence of response after long-term therapy. J Allergy Clin Immunol 2017;140(1):162–9.e2.

24. Menzella F, Galeone C, Formisano D, et al. Real-life efficacy of omalizumab after 9 years of follow-up. Allergy Asthma Immunol Res 2017;9(4):368–72.

25. NUCALA (mepolizumab) prescribing information. Available at. http://www.nucala. com/. Accessed October 5, 2017.

26. Pavord ID, Korn S, Howarth P, et al. Mepolizumab for severe eosinophilic asthma (DREAM): a multicentre, double-blind, placebo-controlled trial. Lancet 2012; 380(9842):651–9.

27. Ortega HG, Liu MC, Pavord ID, et al. Mepolizumab treatment in patients with severe eosinophilic asthma. N Engl J Med 2014;371(13):1198–207.

28. Bel EH, Wenzel SE, Thompson PJ, et al. Oral glucocorticoid-sparing effect of mepolizumab in eosinophilic asthma. N Engl J Med 2014;371(13):1189–97.

29. Wechsler ME, Akuthota P, Jayne D, et al. Mepolizumab or placebo for eosinophilic granulomatosis with polyangiitis. N Engl J Med 2017;376:1921–32.

30. Eskian M, Khorasanizadeh M, Assa'ad AH, et al. Monoclonal antibodies for treatment of eosinophilic esophagitis. Clin Rev Allergy Immunol 2017. https://doi.org/10.1007/s12016-017-8659-7.

31. Castro M, Zangrilli J, Wechsler ME, et al. Reslizumab for inadequately controlled asthma with elevated blood eosinophil counts: results from two multicentre, parallel, double-blind, randomised, placebo-controlled, phase 3 trials. Lancet Respir Med 2015;3(5):355–66.

32. Corren J, Weinstein S, Janka L, et al. Phase 3 study of reslizumab in patients with poorly controlled asthma: effects across a broad range of eosinophil counts. Chest 2016;150(4):799–810.

33. Bleecker ER, FitzGerald JM, Chanez P, et al. Efficacy and safety of benralizumab for patients with severe asthma uncontrolled with high-dosage inhaled corticosteroids and long-acting beta2-agonists (SIROCCO): a randomised, multicentre, placebo-controlled phase 3 trial. Lancet 2016;388(10056):2115–27.

34. FitzGerald JM, Bleecker ER, Nair P, et al. Benralizumab, an anti-interleukin-5 receptor alpha monoclonal antibody, as add-on treatment for patients with severe, uncontrolled, eosinophilic asthma (CALIMA): a randomised, double-blind, placebo-controlled phase 3 trial. Lancet 2016;388(10056):2128–41.

35. Nair P, Wenzel S, Rabe KF, et al. Oral glucocorticoid-sparing effect of benralizumab in severe asthma. N Engl J Med 2017;376(25):2448–58.

36. Nowak RM, Parker JM, Silverman RA, et al. A randomized trial of benralizumab, an antiinterleukin 5 receptor alpha monoclonal antibody, after acute asthma. Am J Emerg Med 2015;33(1):14–20.

37. Farne HA, Wilson A, Powell C, et al. Anti-IL5 therapies for asthma. Cochrane Database Syst Rev 2017;(9):CD010834.

38. Valtrella A, Fabozzi I, Calabrese C, et al. Dupilumab: a novel treatment for asthma. J Asthma Allergy 2014;7:123–30.

39. Castro M, Corren J, Pavord ID, et al. Dupilumab efficacy and safety in moderate-to-severe uncontrolled asthma. N Engl J Med 2018;378:2486–96.

40. Rabe KF, Nair P, Brusselle G, et al. Efficacy and safety of dupilumab in glucocorticoid-dependent severe asthma. N Engl J Med 2018;378:2475–85.

41. Hanania NA, Korenblat P, Chapman KR, et al. Efficacy and safety of lebrikizumab in patients with uncontrolled asthma (LAVOLTA I and LAVOLTA II): replicate, phase 3, randomised, double-blind, placebo-controlled trials. Lancet Respir Med 2016;4(10):781–96.

42. Panettieri RA Jr, Sjobring U, Peterffy A, et al. Tralokinumab for severe, uncontrolled asthma (STRATOS 1 and STRATOS 2): two randomised, double-blind, placebo-controlled, phase 3 clinical trials. Lancet Respir Med 2018;6:511–25.

43. ClinicalTrials.gov. Study to evaluate tezepelumab in adults & adolescents with severe uncontrolled asthma (NAVIGATOR). 2017. Available at: ClinicalTrials.gov.

44. ClinicalTrials.gov. Study to evaluate the efficacy and safety of tezepelumab in reducing oral corticosteroid use in adults with oral corticosteroid dependent asthma (SOURCE). 2018. Available at: https://clinicaltrials.gov/ct2/show/NCT03406078.

45. Arima M, Fukuda T. Prostaglandin D2 and T(H)2 inflammation in the pathogenesis of bronchial asthma. Korean J Intern Med 2011;26(1):8–18.

46. Chevalier E, Stock J, Fisher T, et al. Cutting edge: chemoattractant receptor-homologous molecule expressed on Th2 cells plays a restricting role on IL-5 production and eosinophil recruitment. J Immunol 2005;175(4):2056–60.

47. Erpenbeck VJ, Vets E, Gheyle L, et al. Pharmacokinetics, safety, and tolerability of fevipiprant (QAW039), a novel CRTh2 receptor antagonist: results from 2

randomized, phase 1, placebo-controlled studies in healthy volunteers. Clin Pharmacol Drug Dev 2016;5(4):306–13.

48. Gonem S, Berair R, Singapuri A, et al. Fevipiprant, a prostaglandin D2 receptor 2 antagonist, in patients with persistent eosinophilic asthma: a single-centre, randomised, double-blind, parallel-group, placebo controlled trial. Lancet Respir Med 2016;4(9):699–707.

49. Berry MA, Hargadon B, Shelley M, et al. Evidence of a role of tumor necrosis factor alpha in refractory asthma. N Engl J Med 2006;354:697–708.

50. Holgate ST, Noonan M, Chanez P, et al. Efficacy and safety of etanercept in moderate-to-severe asthma: a randomised, controlled trial. Eur Respir J 2011; 37:1352–9.

51. Kirsten A, Watz H, Pedersen F, et al. The anti-IL-17A antibody secukinumab does not attenuate ozone-induced airway neutrophilia in healthy volunteers. Eur Respir J 2013;41:239–41.

52. Busse WW, Holgate S, Kerwin E, et al. Randomized, double-blind, placebo-controlled study of brodalumab, a human anti-IL-17 receptor monoclonal antibody, in moderate to severe asthma. Am J Respir Crit Care Med 2013;188: 1294–302.

53. Essilfie AT, Horvat JC, Kim RY, et al. Macrolide therapy suppresses key features of experimental steroid-sensitive and steroid-insensitive asthma. Thorax 2015;70: 458–67.

54. Castro M, Rubin AS, Laviolette M, et al, AIR2 Trial Study Group. Effectiveness and safety of bronchial thermoplasty in the treatment of severe asthma: a multicenter, randomized, double-blind, sham-controlled clinical trial. Am J Respir Crit Care Med 2010;181(2):116–24.

55. Trivedi A, Pavord ID, Castro M. Bronchial thermoplasty and biological therapy as targeted treatments for severe uncontrolled asthma. Lancet Respir Med 2016; 4(7):585–92.

56. Wechsler ME, Laviolette M, Rubi AS, et al. Bronchial thermoplasty: long term safety and effectiveness in patients with severe persistent asthma. J Allergy Clin Immunol 2013;132:1295–302.

57. Ohta S, Oda N, Yokoe T, et al. Effect of tiotropium bromide on airway inflammation and remodeling in a mouse model of asthma. Clin Exp Allergy 2010;40:1226–75.

58. Casale TB, Bateman ED, Vanderwalker M, et al. Tiotropium respimat add-on is efficacious in symptomatic asthma, independent of T2 phenotype. J Allergy Clin Immunol 2018;6:923–35.

59. Zafari Z, Sadatsafavi M, Mark FitzGerald J. Cost-effectiveness of tiotropium versus omalizumab for uncontrolled allergic asthma in US. Cost Eff Resour Alloc 2018;16:1.

Diagnosis and Management of Food Allergy

Roxanne Carbonell Oriel, MD, Julie Wang, MD*

KEYWORDS

- Food allergy • Diagnosis • Skin prick test • Allergen-specific serum IgE
- Oral food challenge • Disease management • Anaphylaxis • Prevention

KEY POINTS

- Accurately diagnosing food allergy is critical because significant dietary restrictions and impairment in quality of life for patients and their families can occur.
- Diagnosis requires a compelling clinical history, positive skin prick testing, positive allergen-specific serum immunoglobulin E, and/or oral food challenge.
- Management of food allergies includes allergen avoidance, recognition of signs and symptoms of allergic reactions, and readily available emergency medications to treat reactions.
- There are emerging diagnostic and treatment modalities for food allergies that are very promising.

INTRODUCTION

Food allergy is a growing public health concern given its increasing incidence in infants and children in the last few decades worldwide, particularly in industrialized countries.[1] The most common food allergens are milk, egg, soy, wheat, peanut, tree nuts, fish, and shellfish.[2,3] Seeds, with sesame being the most common, are also increasingly identified as allergens.[4]

Definitions

An adverse food reaction is defined as any abnormal clinical response associated with ingestion of a food. This definition includes both immune-mediated (allergic) and non–immune-mediated mechanisms. Food allergy is defined as an adverse health effect that is caused by a specific immune response and occurs reproducibly on exposure to a given food.[3] Although different conditions come under the term food allergy, the unifying mechanism in the diagnosis is the failure of tolerance to an otherwise benign

Disclosure: The authors have nothing to disclose.
Department of Pediatrics, Division of Allergy & Immunology, Icahn School of Medicine at Mount Sinai, One Gustave L. Levy Place, Box 1198, New York, NY 10029, USA
* Corresponding author.
E-mail address: julie.wang@mssm.edu

Pediatr Clin N Am 66 (2019) 941–954
https://doi.org/10.1016/j.pcl.2019.06.002
0031-3955/19/© 2019 Elsevier Inc. All rights reserved.

exposure to food. **Fig. 1** shows a classification of adverse food reactions based on mechanism.

Food allergy may be categorized in the following way:

- Immunoglobulin (Ig) E mediated: acute urticaria, oral allergy syndrome, anaphylaxis, food-dependent exercise-induced anaphylaxis
- Non–IgE mediated: atopic dermatitis, food protein–induced enterocolitis syndrome, food protein–induced allergic proctocolitis, food protein–induced enteropathy, allergic contact dermatitis, food-induced pulmonary hemosiderosis (Heiner syndrome)
- Mixed IgE mediated and non–IgE mediated: eosinophilic esophagitis or other eosinophilic gastrointestinal disease

For the purposes of this article, food allergy refers to IgE-mediated mechanisms.

Pathophysiology

IgE-mediated allergy to food entails allergen binding to specific IgE antibodies leading to cross-linking of IgE receptors on mast cells and basophils, which trigger the release of preformed mediators, including histamine, tryptase, and chymase, as well as de novo synthesis of leukotrienes, prostaglandins, and platelet-activating factor. These mediators and others are responsible for the symptoms that arise in an allergic reaction: vasodilation leading to erythema, increased permeability of the vasculature yielding swelling, nociceptive nerve activation that is responsible for itching, and smooth muscle constriction that results in bronchoconstriction and abdominal pain.

Clinical Manifestations

IgE-mediated food allergy reactions manifest with acute symptoms involving skin, respiratory tract, gastrointestinal tract, and/or the cardiovascular system, usually minutes to a few hours after ingestion of the culprit food protein. **Table 1** lists symptoms

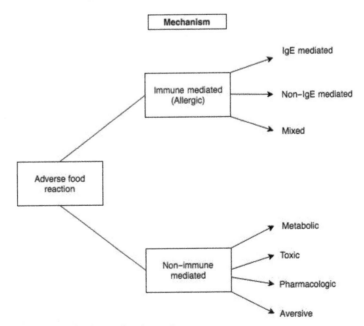

Fig. 1. Classification of adverse food reactions.

Table 1	
Symptoms of an immunoglobulin E–mediated allergic reaction	
Cutaneous	Urticaria, angioedema, pruritus, flushing, morbilliform rash
Respiratory	Upper airway: rhinorrhea, nasal pruritus, nasal congestion, sneezing, hoarseness, stridor Lower airway: cough, wheeze, dyspnea, cyanosis
Cardiovascular	Increased heart rate, low blood pressure, pallor, dizziness, shock, loss of consciousness
Gastrointestinal	Swelling of lips/tongue/uvula, nausea, vomiting, abdominal cramps, diarrhea
Neurologic	Anxiety, headache, seizure, altered mental status, feeling of impending doom
Ocular	Conjunctival erythema and tearing

suggestive of an IgE-mediated reaction. A diagnosis of food allergy should be suspected if allergic symptoms occur shortly after ingesting a food, particularly if symptoms have reproducibly followed ingestion of the given food on more than 1 occasion. One noteworthy exception is alpha-gal allergy, which is an IgE-mediated reaction to meats following sensitization to a carbohydrate antigen from a tick bite. In this type of allergy, symptoms are usually delayed and occur 4 to 6 hours after ingestion.

Epidemiology

The prevalence of food allergy differs in various parts of the world and varies depending on the allergen in question. Prevalence estimates are difficult to ascertain because the gold standard for determining diagnosis is a double-blind, placebo-controlled oral food challenge (DBPCFC), but many epidemiologic studies estimate prevalence based on self-reported food allergy or sensitization only (ie, positive skin prick test [SPT] and/or allergen-specific serum IgE [sIgE]).

In the population-based HealthNuts study conducted in Australia, infants underwent skin prick testing and an oral food challenge if the wheal size was greater than or equal to 1 mm to raw egg, peanut, and/or sesame. More than 10% of infants showed food challenge–confirmed allergies at age 1 year to 1 or more foods.[5] In a follow-up study with additional recruitment of subjects, the prevalence of challenge-confirmed food allergy to any food at age 4 years was 3.8%, with resolution of egg allergy largely responsible for the decrease in prevalence.[6] In the EuroPrevall birth cohort, the prevalence of challenge-proven food allergy in the first 2 years of life was 0.59% for milk and 1.23% for egg.[7,8] **Table 2** lists prevalence data from around the world based on challenge-proven food allergy.

In contrast with studies performed in other industrialized nations, the US food allergy prevalence data evaluated broader age ranges but relied on self-report or sensitization, which likely overestimate true prevalence. Using several surveys, including the National Health Interview Survey and the National Health and Nutrition Examination Survey, Branum and Lukacs[9] suggest that approximately 5% of children less than 5 years of age and 4% of adolescents and adults are affected by food allergy. In a more recent study using a population-based survey completed via Web or telephone between 2015 and 2016, food allergy prevalence in children in the United States was estimated at 7.6%.[10] A study conducted by the same group found that food allergy prevalence in children was 8.0% based on an electronic survey distributed between 2009 and 2010.[11] The investigators note that a direct comparison

Table 2 Prevalence of challenge-proven food allergy				
	Peanut (%)	Egg (%)	Sesame (%)	Milk (%)
HealthNuts (Australia)				
Peters et al[6] Age 1 y	3.1	9.5	0.6	—
Peters et al[6] Age 4 y	1.9	1.2	0.4	—
EuroPrevall (Europe)				
Schoemaker et al[7] Up to age 2 y	—	—	—	0.59
Xepapadaki et al[8] Up to age 2 y	—	1.23	—	—
South Africa				
Botha et al[66] 1–3 y	0.8	1.9	—	0.1
China				
Chen et al[67] 0–12 mo	—	2.5	—	1.3

between the 2 studies cannot be drawn given stricter criteria used in the diagnosis of food allergy in the more recent study.

Natural History

Although many with food allergy outgrow this condition, the natural course of the disease differs depending on the allergen, with most outgrowing milk, egg, wheat, and/or soy allergies and those with peanut, tree nut, fish, and/or shellfish allergies tending to have lifelong allergy.[12] Predictors of persistent food allergy include more severe initial reaction characteristics, presence of other food allergy or other allergic conditions (atopic dermatitis, asthma, or allergic rhinitis), increased severity of comorbid conditions, earlier age at diagnosis, lower eliciting dose for reaction, larger SPT wheal size, and higher allergen-specific sIgE level.[13–17] The rate of decline in SPT wheal size and sIgE level over time is informative in assessing food allergy resolution.

DIAGNOSIS

Given the potential social and nutritional impact of food avoidances, correctly diagnosing patients with food allergy is paramount. Establishing a diagnosis of food allergy involves a careful clinical history, evidence of allergen-specific IgE by skin and/or blood testing, and in some cases an oral food challenge. Although new diagnostic tools are being developed, such as the basophil activation test, these approaches will require validation and standardization before they become available for use in routine clinical practice.

Clinical History

The most important tool in establishing a diagnosis of IgE-mediated food allergy is an accurate allergy-focused clinical history. However, history alone is not enough to establish a definitive diagnosis of food allergy and this can only be confirmed by a positive DBPCFC in approximately 30% to 40% of individuals.[3,18,19] Specific inquiry should be undertaken for foods ingested with specific characteristics (raw vs heated), amount of food ingested, time course between ingestion and symptom onset, manifested symptoms, outcomes of prior exposure to the food, and possible potentiating factors (ie, alcohol, exercise). Whether the patient has had the food following initial reaction with recurrence of symptoms should also be noted. If subsequent exposure has occurred without symptoms, then an alternative culprit food or diagnosis should be sought. Other questions for the patient and caregiver include the treatment following reaction and the length of time that has elapsed since ingestion with or without allergic reaction. Careful history taking allows the health care provider to discern whether the clinical picture is concerning for an IgE-mediated reaction.

Comorbid atopic conditions should also be noted, including atopic dermatitis, asthma, allergic rhinitis, and eosinophilic gastrointestinal disease. Children with atopic dermatitis are at greatest risk for food allergy.[20,21] Particular attention should be given to the presence or absence of atopic dermatitis, with age of onset and severity noted, because more than 50% of infants developing severe eczema in the first few months of life develop IgE-mediated allergy to foods.[22]

Skin Prick Test

SPTs with commercially available extracts provide an immediate method to screen patients for the presence of food-specific IgE antibodies bound to mast cells in the skin. The technique is a simple, inexpensive, and reproducible in vivo test that involves a drop of allergen to the volar surface of the arm followed by a small skin prick using a skin prick testing device (multiple types are commercially available). After 10 to 15 minutes, the wheal site is measured. Important considerations when evaluating skin test results include that commercial extracts and methods of performing and recording SPT results lack standardization. Furthermore, variations between devices have been shown, with increased histamine concentrations required for less sensitive devices and mean wheal diameters differing depending on device used.[23]

A wheal of 3 mm or greater than the negative control is considered positive. Although SPT has a poor positive predictive value, it has a high negative predictive value. Therefore, SPT is useful for ruling out food allergy.[19] The size of the SPT wheal correlates with the likelihood of food allergy, with larger sizes indicating a higher risk of clinical allergy.[17,24] Specifically, with cow's milk, hen's egg, or peanut, wheal diameters greater than 8 mm were greater than 95% predictive of clinical reactivity to the specific food.[25] Multiple studies have shown that there is no reliable correlation between wheal size and severity of reaction.[20]

Positive SPT represents food sensitization, so a positive test in the absence of a clinical history suggestive of allergy is not diagnostic, thus testing should be pursued in the context of high clinical suspicion for allergy.

If the clinical history is suggestive of a food allergy, but the diagnostic testing is negative, then oral food challenge may need to be performed to definitively diagnose or eliminate the diagnosis. False-negative skin test results can occur in cases in which the allergen is not present in sufficient quantities in the commercial extract. In these cases, skin-prick testing with fresh foods may helpful, in particular with fruits and vegetables because the extract manufacturing process can denature the relevant allergens. This technique is not standardized and irritant reactions to the fresh food may occur.[26]

Allergen-specific Serum Immunoglobulin E Test

sIgE testing is an in vitro immunoassay in which allergen is covalently coupled to a solid phase and binds with the specific IgE in the patient's serum sample. Results are typically reported in allergen-specific kilounits (kU_A) per liter. Like SPT, a positive test indicates sensitization to a food, but in itself is not diagnostic of clinical allergy. In

Table 3
Predictive values for food allergen–specific immunoglobulin E (kU$_A$/L) and skin prick test wheal size (millimeters)

	Milk	Egg	Soy	Wheat	Peanut	Tree Nuts	Fish
Likely Reactive if ≥	15 (95%) ≤2 y: 5 (95%) SPT: ≥8 (95%)[20]	7 (98%) ≤2 y: 2 (95%) SPT: ≥7 (95%)[20]	65	80	14 (100%) 1 y: 34 (95%) 4 y: 2.1 SPT: ≥8 (95%)[20,65]	15 (95%)	20 (100%)
Possibly Reactive	—	SPT ≤3 (50%)[20]	30 (73%)	26 (74%)	SPT ≤3 (50%)[20]	—	—
Unlikely Reactive if <	0.35	0.35	0.35	0.35	0.35	0.35	0.35

Positive predictive values are indicated in parentheses.
Adapted from Sampson HA. Utility of food-specific IgE concentrations in predicting symptomatic food allergy. JACI 2001;107:891-6. Other references are noted in the table or text.

addition, sIgE may be undetectable to a food that triggers clinical allergy, so a compelling history and a negative sIgE warrants further evaluation. In cases such as these, additional evaluation with SPT and/or oral food challenge can be informative.

Similar to SPT, increasing concentration of food-specific IgE correlates with an increased risk of clinical allergy, but the level of sIgE does not accurately predict the severity of allergic reactions that can be triggered by the allergen.[3] Clinical decision points have been published for some major food allergens and these can be found in **Table 3**. Considerations when applying these positive predictive values to clinical practice include age, population studied, comorbid conditions, and clinical history.[27–32]

Periodic testing with SPT and/or sIgE should be performed to reevaluate food allergy status because some individuals have transient allergy.

Component-resolved Diagnostics

Component-resolved diagnostics (CRD) refers to sIgE testing that is directed toward specific food antigens or epitopes. Testing for specific epitopes can increase specificity by distinguishing clinically relevant IgE from IgE directed at nonallergic components. This approach is in contrast with conventional testing, which measures IgE to whole food extracts that contain multiple proteins. An example of the potential benefit of CRD is in patients with birch pollen allergy who may have detectable IgE to whole peanut extract because of cross-reactivity (Bet v 1 of birch pollen is homologous with Ara h 8 of peanut). Monosensitization to Ara h 8 predicts tolerance to peanut.[33] Ara h 2 and Ara h 6, other peanut allergens, not only have the highest diagnostic accuracy for peanut allergy but also can help approximate the severity of allergy. In a prospective study in peanut-allergic patients aged 6 to 18 years, sensitization to the most potent peanut allergens Ara h 2 or Ara h 6 was 100% sensitive for moderate or severe peanut allergy, with Ara h 6 the best marker for moderate or severe allergy.[34] Furthermore, polysensitization to Ara h 1, Ara h 2, and Ara h 3 was 100% specific for moderate or severe peanut allergy.[34] CRD for several major food allergens are commercially available (**Table 4**); however, questions remain regarding clinically relevant cutoff values and cost-effectiveness of additional diagnostic testing.[35]

Table 4
Major food allergens and their component proteins

Food	Component Protein	Clinical Relevance
Cow's milk	Bos d8 (casein)	Increased levels of casein indicate increased likelihood of reactivity to extensively heated milk
Egg	Gal d1 (ovomucoid)	Increased levels of ovomucoid indicate increased likelihood of reactivity to extensively heated egg
Peanut	Ara h1	Associated with systemic reactivity
	Ara h2	Associated with systemic reactivity
	Ara h3	Associated with systemic reactivity
	Ara h6	Associated with systemic reactivity
	Ara h8	Cross-reactive with Bet v1 (birch pollen). In absence of other component proteins or if predominant component, usually indicates clinical tolerance or predictive of only mild oral allergy symptoms
	Ara h9	Associated with systemic reactivity (Mediterranean populations)
Hazelnut	Cor a1	Cross-reactive with Bet v1 (birch pollen). In absence of other component proteins or if predominant component, usually indicates clinical tolerance or predictive of only mild oral allergy symptoms
	Cor a8	Associated with systemic reactivity (Mediterranean populations)
	Cor a9	Associated with systemic reactivity
	Cor a14	Associated with systemic reactivity
Cashew	Ana o3	Associated with systemic reactivity
Walnut	Jug r1	Associated with systemic reactivity

Oral Food Challenge

This procedure is the most definitive means to diagnose a food allergy. Oral food challenges entail supervised ingestion of increasing amounts of the suspected food allergen over a defined period of time with subsequent monitoring in an office or hospital setting with personnel equipped to treat an allergic reaction. The gold standard for diagnosis is a DBPCFC. Because this is a time-consuming and resource-intensive procedure, open food challenge or a single-blind challenge may be considered instead. When no symptoms occur during challenge, it is referred to as a negative challenge and recommendations to incorporate the food into the diet are advised. When objective or persistent subjective symptoms are observed, this is referred to as a positive challenge and confirms a diagnosis of allergy.

Different protocols for performing oral food challenges are available and may vary based on age of the patient, food (raw, cooked, or baked), dosing amounts, and time intervals between doses.[36,37]

Testing that Has No Proven Utility

A multitude of tests are available and purported to aid in diagnosis of food allergy. However, the following tests have no proven benefit: IgG testing, applied kinesiology, hair analysis, electrodermal test, facial thermography, gastric juice analysis, endoscopic allergen provocation.[38]

Future of Diagnostics

The basophil histamine release/activation test (BAT) has the potential to discriminate patients with clinical reactivity versus sensitization to foods by mimicking what occurs in vivo. As mentioned, a food allergic reaction occurs when an ingested food antigen interacts with IgE and its high-affinity Fc receptor (FcεRI) on the surface membrane of mast cells in mucosal tissues and on circulating basophils. Subsequent FcεRI cross-linking leads to release of histamine and other preformed mediators. The BAT measures markers of basophil activation, cluster of differentiation (CD) 63 and CD203c expression, by flow cytometry following allergen stimulation of a patient's basophils in vitro. This testing might be useful in the future as an intermediate step before proceeding with an oral food challenge if the SPT and sIgE are equivocal.[39,40]

The mast cell activation test is another promising diagnostic tool currently used in research. A patient's allergen-specific IgE antibodies are used to elicit mast cell degranulation. This test may also prove useful as an intermediate step to differentiate allergy versus sensitization. Recent studies have shown increased specificity when using this test to diagnose peanut allergy.[41,42]

MANAGEMENT

The current management recommendations for individuals with food allergy remain strict avoidance of the allergen and preparation to manage allergic reactions in case of accidental exposures. Successful food allergen avoidance entails reading ingredient labels and knowledge of cross-contact/cross-contamination issues. However, allergen avoidance is not always infallible and allergic reactions can occur that are unpredictable, ranging from mild to severe. Therefore, patients are prescribed epinephrine autoinjectors to have emergency medication available at all times.

Age and developmentally appropriate management guidance should be provided to families. Management of infants and young children with food allergy is particularly difficult because they are unable to recognize or verbalize allergy symptoms. In addition, infants and young children explore the world using their mouths. As such, they frequently place objects such as toys and hands in their mouths, which can lead to allergen exposure outside of mealtimes. Adolescents are at particularly high risk for allergic reactions because of nonadherence to recommended strategies for avoidance and riskier behaviors, including intentional exposures and not having an epinephrine autoinjector readily available.[43–45]

Allergen Labeling

Several countries have enacted legislation mandating allergen labeling on packaged goods for the most common food allergens to improve safety for food allergy consumers.[46] In 2004, the US Congress passed the Food Allergen Labeling and Consumer Protection Act, which required listing milk, egg, soy, wheat, peanut, tree nuts, fish, and crustacean shellfish on packaged goods. This legislative action also required that the allergen be listed in unambiguous terms (ie, label must include milk in addition to casein, whey). Similar legislation passed in Europe in 2014 and required the following allergens to be listed: milk, egg, gluten, lupine, soy, peanut, tree nuts, sesame seed, mustard seed, fish, crustacean and mollusk shellfish, celery and celeriac, and sulfur dioxide and sulfites. Several other countries have allergen labeling legislation as well, with variations in terms of which allergens are covered (https://farrp.unl.edu/IRChart).

Precautionary advisory labeling (PAL) uses phrases that include "may contain [allergen]," "processed in a facility that manufactures [allergen]," or "manufactured on shared equipment with [allergen]" and appears on 17% of manufactured products in the United States and on 65% of products in Australia.[47,48] Patients should be educated that PAL is unregulated and not mandated by law, but is pervasive on packaged goods. PAL often leads to consumer confusion because these labels do not reliably correspond with the presence or absence of detectable allergenic proteins.[49]

Anaphylaxis

Management of anaphylaxis entails prompt recognition and management. Studies have shown that early use of epinephrine leads to improved anaphylaxis outcomes (both morbidity and mortality).[50,51] When counseling patients, it is key to discuss that reaction severity and the threshold dose of allergen to trigger allergic reactions is unpredictable and although cutaneous manifestations such as urticaria and pruritus are common, these symptoms may be absent in up to 20% of patients who have anaphylaxis.[52] Patients should be provided prescriptions for epinephrine autoinjectors and trained on how the devices should be used. In addition, written allergy and anaphylaxis emergency plans that outline signs and symptoms of allergic reactions and indications for use of emergency medications should be provided (www.aap.org/anaphylaxis) and updated at least annually or whenever medical changes occur.[53]

PREVENTION

Given the increasing prevalence of food allergy in infants and children, strategies for prevention have been explored. In the Learning Early About Peanut (LEAP) trial, investigators found that, among infants at high risk for allergy, sustained consumption of peanut resulted in an 81% lower rate of peanut allergy.[54] In the follow-up Persistence of Oral Tolerance to Peanut (LEAP-On) study, peanut tolerance caused by early peanut consumption was maintained despite peanut avoidance for 12 months.[55] These landmark studies led a transformational shift to now encouraging and supporting early peanut introduction into the diets of high-risk infants. The National Institute of Allergy and Infectious Diseases–sponsored expert panel published guidelines on recommendations for patients with severe eczema, egg allergy, or both.[56] Patients with peanut IgE level less than 0.35 kU_A/L and/or peanut SPT of 0 to 2 mm should either introduce peanut at home or have a supervised feeding in office. Peanut IgE level greater than or equal to 0.35 kU_A/L should have further evaluation by an allergist. For patients with peanut SPT of 3 to 7 mm, a supervised feeding in office or graded oral food challenge should be offered. In addition, for patients with SPT greater than or equal to 8 mm, current recommendations are to strictly avoid peanut because of likely peanut allergy. For lower risk infants, those with mild to moderate eczema, peanut-containing foods should be introduced around 6 months of age. For infants without eczema or any food allergy, the current recommendation is to introduce peanut-containing foods when age appropriate and in line with family preferences. In a meta-analysis evaluating the effect of early introduction of egg between the ages of 4 and 6 months, introduction to the diet was associated with lower risk of egg allergy.[57] Other ongoing studies are examining the potential benefits of early introduction of other highly allergenic foods.

Other approaches are being investigated for prevention. Atopic dermatitis is frequently found as a comorbid condition in children with food allergy and there is evidence to support that food allergen exposure through the impaired skin barrier rather than through oral exposure leads to a failure of tolerance in the gastrointestinal tract.[58] In an ongoing clinical trial in the United Kingdom (Barrier Enhancement for Eczema Prevention [BEEP] study), investigators are assessing the effect of daily application of emollients in the first year of life and risk of development of atopic dermatitis.[59] In another study currently enrolling patients, conducted by the Immune Tolerance Network and sponsored by the National Institute of Allergy and Infectious Diseases, investigators are seeking to assess the early influence of vaginal microbiome exposure in cesarean section infants and risk of allergen sensitization at 1 year of age (ClinicalTrials.gov identifier: NCT03567707).

TREATMENTS FOR FOOD ALLERGY

Several treatment approaches are currently being explored for food allergies, with recent clinical trials focusing on oral, epicutaneous, and sublingual immunotherapies. Clinical trials have focused on desensitization, which refers to increasing the threshold dose of allergen to trigger allergic reactions while on therapy. Few studies have assessed for sustained unresponsiveness, which is defined as a lack of responsiveness to a food after immunotherapy has been discontinued.

Oral immunotherapy (OIT) entails incremental ingestion of increasing doses of allergen, with the aim of desensitization to protect allergic individuals from accidental allergen exposure. This daily treatment approach has been most extensively studied for peanut. The largest study to date show that 67.2% of children and adolescents aged 4 to 17 years who are highly allergic to peanut (ie, dose-limiting symptoms of 100 mg or less of peanut protein) who received an investigational oral immunotherapy drug were able to ingest 600 mg of protein or more when maintained on 300 mg of peanut protein for 6 months.[60] Side effects of OIT include allergic reactions, ranging from mild to severe, as well as persistent gastrointestinal symptoms, which have raised concerns for eosinophilic esophagitis. Areas requiring further investigation include whether sustained unresponsiveness is possible, long-term outcomes of OIT, and biomarkers to identify patients who would benefit from OIT. Ongoing studies are examining OIT for other allergens as well as a combination of allergens.

Epicutaneous immunotherapy (EPIT) has been studied for peanut and milk allergy. EPIT involves exposure of the cutaneous immune system to the allergen, with the goal of offering protection against accidental allergen exposures. Based on outcomes reported to date, there seems to be minimal risk to patients with this approach; only mild skin irritation at the patch site has been noted in most subjects in clinical trials. In a recently completed phase 3 trial in children 4 to 11 years of age evaluating the efficacy of a 250-μg transdermal peanut patch, 35.6% in the active group versus 13.6% in the placebo group were responders ($P<.0001$).[61] Responders were defined as tolerating greater than or equal to 300 mg of the eliciting dose (ED) with baseline ED less than or equal to 10 mg, or an ED greater than or equal to 1000 mg.

Sublingual immunotherapy (SLIT) requires administration of food allergen extract under the tongue, with doses ranging from 2 to 7 mg of protein. With this approach, desensitization can be achieved after 1 year of treatment.[62,63] However, note that these were small clinical trials evaluating the efficacy of SLIT. This approach has a favorable safety profile, with side effects primarily limited to oropharyngeal itching and tingling.

A robust pipeline of other food allergy therapies are undergoing study, including use of biologics, vaccines using modified proteins or DNA, probiotics, Chinese herbal formulas, and combination therapies.[64,65]

SUMMARY

IgE-mediated food allergy is a global health problem affecting multiple facets of these patients' lives. Therefore, correctly diagnosing these patients is paramount. The diagnostic approach includes a detailed clinical history, SPT, sIgE, and/or oral food challenge, and management involves strict avoidance of foods as well as preparedness to treat allergic reactions. The field of food allergy is rapidly advancing because many emerging diagnostic tools and potential treatments are on their way to clinical practice. Research is also ongoing to develop preventive strategies for food allergy.

REFERENCES

1. Renz H, Allen KJ, Sicherer SH, et al. Food allergy. Nat Rev Dis Primers 2018;4: 17098.
2. Sicherer SH, Sampson HA. Food allergy: a review and update on epidemiology, pathogenesis, diagnosis, prevention, and management. J Allergy Clin Immunol 2018;141(1):41–58.
3. Boyce J, Assa'ad A, Burks AW, et al. Guidelines for the diagnosis and management of food allergy in the United States: report of the NIAID-sponsored expert panel. J Allergy Clin Immunol 2010;125(6Suppl):S1–58.
4. Patel A, Bahna SL. Hypersensitivities to sesame and other common edible seeds. Allergy 2016;71(10):1405–13.
5. Osborne NJ, Koplin JJ, Martin PE, et al, HealthNuts Investigators. Prevalence of challenge-proven IgE-mediated food allergy using population-based sampling and predetermined challenge criteria in infants. J Allergy Clin Immunol 2011; 127(3):668–76.
6. Peters RL, Koplin JJ, Gurrin LC, et al, HealthNuts Study. The prevalence of food allergy and other allergic diseases in early childhood in a population-based study: HealthNuts age 4-year follow-up. J Allergy Clin Immunol 2017;140(1): 145–53.
7. Schoemaker AA, Sprikkelman AB, Grimshaw KE, et al. Incidence and natural history of challenge-proven cow's milk allergy in European children -EuroPrevall birth cohort. Allergy 2015;70:963–72.
8. Xepapadaki P, Fiocchi A, Grabenhenrich L, et al. Incidence and natural history of hen's egg allergy in the first 2 years of life - the EuroPrevall birth cohort study. Allergy 2016;71:350–7.
9. Branum AM, Lukacs SL. Food allergy among children in the United States. Pediatrics 2009;124(6):1549–55.
10. Gupta RS, Warren CM, Smith BM, et al. The public health impact of parent-reported childhood food allergies in the United States. Pediatrics 2018;142(6): e20181235.
11. Gupta RS, Springston EE, Warrier MR, et al. The prevalence, severity, and distribution of childhood food allergy in the United States. Pediatrics 2011;128(1): e9–17.
12. Savage J, Sicherer S, Wood R. The natural history of food allergy. J Allergy Clin Immunol Pract 2016;4:196–203.
13. Sicherer SH, Wood RA, Vickery BP, et al. The natural history of egg allergy in an observational cohort. J Allergy Clin Immunol 2014;133(2):492–9.
14. Spergel JM, Beausoleil JL, Pawlowski NA. Resolution of childhood peanut allergy. Ann Allergy Asthma Immunol 2000;85(6 Pt 1):473–6.

15. Boyano-Martínez T, García-Ara C, Díaz-Pena JM, et al. Prediction of tolerance on the basis of quantification of egg white-specific IgE antibodies in children with egg allergy. J Allergy Clin Immunol 2002;110(2):304–9.

16. Elizur A, Rajuan N, Goldberg MR, et al. Natural course and risk factors for persistence of IgE-mediated cow's milk allergy. J Pediatr 2012;161(3):482–7.

17. Savage JH, Matsui EC, Skripak JM, et al. The natural history of egg allergy. J Allergy Clin Immunol 2007;120(6):1413–7.

18. Sampson HA, Aceves S, Bock SA, et al. Food allergy. A practice parameter update – 2014. J Allergy Clin Immunol 2014;134:1016–25.e43.

19. Sampson HA. Food allergy – accurately identifying clinical reactivity. Allergy 2005;60(Suppl. 79):19–24.

20. Genuneit J, Seibold AM, Apfelbacher CJ, et al. Overview of systematic reviews in allergy epidemiology. Allergy 2017;72:849–56.

21. Du Toit G, Tsakok T, Lack S, et al. Prevention of food allergy. J Allergy Clin Immunol 2016;137:998–1010.

22. Martin PE, Eckert JK, Koplin JJ, et al. Which infants with eczema are at risk of food allergy? Results from a population-based cohort. Clin Exp Allergy 2015;45:255–64.

23. Tversky JR, Chelladurai Y, McGready J, et al. Performance and pain tolerability of current diagnostic allergy skin prick test devices. J Allergy Clin Immunol Pract 2015;3(6):888–93.

24. Peters RL, Gurrin LC, Allen KJ, et al. The predictive value of skin prick testing for challenge-proven food allergy: a systematic review. Pediatr Allergy Immunol 2012;23(4):347–52.

25. Sporik R, Hill DJ, Hosking CS. Specificity of allergen skin testing in predicting positive open food challenges to milk, egg and peanut in children. Clin Exp Allergy 2000;30(11):1540–6.

26. Nowak-Wegrzyn A, Burks W, Sampson HA. Chapter 81: reactions to foods. In: Middleton E, Franklin Adkinson N, Busse WW, et al, editors. Middleton's allergy: principles and practice, vol. 2, 8th edition. Philadelphia: W B Saunders; 2014. p. 1237–59.

27. Komata T, Soderstrom L, Borres MP, et al. The predictive relationship of food-specific serum IgE concentrations to challenge outcomes for egg and milk varies by patient age. J Allergy Clin Immunol 2007;119(5):1272–4.

28. Maloney JM, Rudengren M, Ahlstedt S, et al. The use of serum-specific IgE measurements for the diagnosis of peanut, tree nut, and seed allergy. J Allergy Clin Immunol 2008;122:145–51.

29. Perry TT, Matsui EC, Kay Conover-Walker M, et al. The relationship of allergen-specific IgE levels and oral food challenge outcome. J Allergy Clin Immunol 2004;114:144–9.

30. Clark AT, Ewan PW. Interpretation of tests for nut allergy in one thousand patients, in relation to allergy or tolerance. Clin Exp Allergy 2003;33:1041–5.

31. Garcia-Ara C, Boyano-Martinez T, Diaz-Pena JM, et al. Specific IgE levels in the diagnosis of immediate hypersensitivity to cow's milk protein in the infant. J Allergy Clin Immunol 2001;107:185–90.

32. Sampson HA. Utility of food-specific IgE concentrations in predicting symptomatic food allergy. J Allergy Clin Immunol 2001;107:891–6.

33. Asarnoj A, Nilsson C, Lidholm J, et al. Peanut component Ara h 8 sensitization and tolerance to peanut. J Allergy Clin Immunol 2012;130:468–72.

34. Kukkonen AK, Pelkonen AS, Makinen-Kiljunen S, et al. Ara h 2 and Ara 6 are the best predictors of severe peanut allergy: a double-blind placebo-controlled study. Allergy 2015;70:1239–45.

35. Kim JF, McCleary N, Nwaru BI, et al. Diagnostic accuracy, risk assessment, and cost-effectiveness of component-resolved diagnostics for food allergy: a systematic review. Allergy 2018;73(8):1609–21.

36. Bird JA, Groetch M, Allen KJ, et al. Conducting an oral food challenge to peanut in an infant. J Allergy Clin Immunol Pract 2017;5(2):301–11.e1.

37. Nowak-Wegrzyn A, Assa'ad AH, Bahna SL, et al. Work group report: oral food challenge testing. adverse reactions to Food Committee of American Academy of Allergy, Asthma & Immunology. J Allergy Clin Immunol 2009;123(6 Suppl): S365–83.

38. Kelso JM. Unproven diagnostic tests for adverse reactions to foods. J Allergy Clin Immunol Pract 2018;6(2):362–5.

39. Hoffmann HJ, Santos AF, Mayorga C, et al. The clinical utility of basophil activation testing in diagnosis and monitoring of allergic disease. Allergy 2015;70(11): 1393–405.

40. Koplin JJ, Perrett KP, Sampson HA. Diagnosing peanut allergy with fewer oral food challenges. J Allergy Clin Immunol Pract 2019;7(2):375–80.

41. Santos AF, Couto-Francisco N, Bécares N, et al. A novel human mast cell activation test for peanut allergy. J Allergy Clin Immunol 2018;142(2):689–91.e9.

42. Bahri R, Custovic A, Korosec P, et al. Mast cell activation test in the diagnosis of allergic disease and anaphylaxis. J Allergy Clin Immunol 2018;142(2):485–96.e16.

43. Smith TD, Camacho J, Wang J. Behavioral risks associated with food allergy management in an urban pediatric population. J Allergy Clin Immunol 2018;6: 680–2.

44. Robinson M, Koplin JJ, Field MJ, et al. Patterns of carriage of prescribed adrenaline autoinjectors in 10- to 14-year-old food-allergic students: a population-based study. J Allergy Clin Immunol Pract 2018;7(2):437–43.

45. Macadam C, Barnett J, Roberts G, et al. What factors affect the carriage of epinephrine auto-injectors by teenagers? Clin Transl Allergy 2012;2:3.

46. Taylor SL, Hefle SL. Food allergen labeling in the USA and Europe. Curr Opin Allergy Clin Immunol 2006;6:186–90.

47. Pieretti MM, Chung D, Pacenza R, et al. Audit of manufactured products: use of allergen advisory labels and identification of labeling ambiguities. J Allergy Clin Immunol 2009;124:337–41.

48. Zurzolo GA, Mathai ML, Koplin JJ, et al. Precautionary allergen labeling following new labeling practice in Australia. J Paediatr Child Health 2013;49:E306–10.

49. Ford LS, Taylor SL, Pacenza R, et al. Food allergen advisory labeling and product contamination with egg, milk, and peanut. J Allergy Clin Immunol 2010;126:384–5.

50. Fleming JT, Clark S, Camargo CA Jr, et al. Early treatment of food-induced anaphylaxis with epinephrine is associated with a lower risk of hospitalization. J Allergy Clin Immunol Pract 2015;3(1):57–62.

51. Hochstadter E, Clarke A, De Schryver S, et al. Increasing visits for anaphylaxis and the benefits of early epinephrine administration: a 4-year study at a pediatric emergency department in Montreal, Canada. J Allergy Clin Immunol Pract 2016; 137(6):1888–90.e4.

52. Arkwright PD, MacMahon J, Koplin J, et al. Severity and threshold of peanut reactivity during hospital-based open oral food challenges: an international multicenter survey. Pediatr Allergy Immunol 2018;29(7):754–61.

53. Wang J, Sicherer SH, American Academy of Pediatrics, Section on Allergy and Immunology. Guidance on completing a written allergy and anaphylaxis emergency plan. Pediatrics 2017;139(3):e20164005.

54. Du Toit G, Roberts G, Sayre PH, et al. Randomized trial of peanut consumption in infants at risk for peanut allergy. N Engl J Med 2015;372(9):803–13.

55. Du Toit G, Sayre PH, Roberts G, et al. Effect of avoidance on peanut allergy after early peanut consumption. N Engl J Med 2016;374:1435–43.

56. Togias A, Cooper SF, Acebal ML, et al. Addendum guidelines for the prevention of peanut allergy in the United States: report of the National Institute of Allergy and Infectious Diseases-sponsored expert panel. J Allergy Clin Immunol 2017; 139(1):29–44.

57. Ierodiakonou D, Garcia-Larsen V, Logan A, et al. Timing of allergenic food introduction to the infant diet and risk of allergic or autoimmune disease: a systematic review and meta-analysis. JAMA 2016;316:1181–92.

58. Brough HA, Liu AH, Sicherer S, et al. Atopic dermatitis increases the effect of exposure to peanut antigen in dust on peanut sensitization and likely peanut allergy. J Allergy Clin Immunol 2015;135:164–70.

59. Chalmers JR, Haines RH, Mitchell EJ, et al. Effectiveness and cost-effectiveness of daily all-over-body application of emollient during the first year of life for preventing atopic eczema in high-risk children (The BEEP trial): protocol for a randomized controlled trial. Trials 2017;18:343.

60. Vickery BP, Vereda A, Casale TB, et al. AR101 oral immunotherapy for peanut allergy. N Engl J Med 2018;379(21):1991–2001.

61. Fleischer DM, Sussman GL, Begin P, et al. Effect of epicutaneous immunotherapy on inducing peanut desensitization in peanut-allergic children: topline peanut epicutaneous immunotherapy efficacy and safety (PEPITES) randomized clinical trial results. J Allergy Clin Immunol 2018;141(2):AB410.

62. Kim EH, Bird JA, Kulis M, et al. Sublingual immunotherapy for peanut allergy: clinical and immunologic evidence of desensitization. J Allergy Clin Immunol 2011; 127(3):640–6.e1.

63. Fleischer DM, Burks AW, Vickery BP, et al. Sublingual immunotherapy for peanut allergy: a randomized, double-blind, placebo-controlled multicenter trial. J Allergy Clin Immunol 2013;131(1):119–27.e1-7.

64. Virkud YV, Wang J, Shreffler WG. Enhancing the safety and efficacy of food allergy immunotherapy: a review of adjunctive therapies. Clin Rev Allergy Immunol 2018;55(2):172–89.

65. Cook QS, Burks AW. Peptide and recombinant allergen vaccines for food allergy. Clin Rev Allergy Immunol 2018;55(2):162–71.

66. Botha M, Basera W, Facey-Thomas HE, et al. Rural and urban food allergy prevalence from the South African Food Allergy (SAFFA) study. J Allergy Clin Immunol 2019;143(2):662–8.e2.

67. Chen J, Hu Y, Allen KJ, et al. The prevalence of food allergy in infants in Chongqing, China. Pediatr Allergy Immunol 2011;22(4):356–60.

Eosinophilic Esophagitis

Heather K. Lehman, MD*, Weyman Lam, MD

KEYWORDS

- Eosinophilic esophagitis • Dysphagia • Food allergy • Eosinophilia • Atopy

KEY POINTS

- Eosinophilic esophagitis is a disease with increasing prevalence over several decades.
- Pediatric and adult eosinophilic esophagitis differ in their clinical presentation, with dysphagia and food impaction being major symptoms for adults, whereas young children present with more vague symptoms.
- Strict elemental diet results in histologic remission in nearly all cases of eosinophilic esophagitis, pointing to the role of food allergy in disease pathogenesis.
- Therapy with topical steroids is effective in the treatment of eosinophilic esophagitis, but disease recurs with discontinuation of therapy.

INTRODUCTION

Eosinophilic esophagitis (EoE) is a disease of the esophagus that is recognized in both children and adults.[1] It is characterized by significant esophageal eosinophilia with severe squamous epithelial hyperplasia generally occurring in association with upper gastrointestinal symptoms.[1] The gastric and duodenal mucosae are not affected. The diagnosis has been traditionally limited to patients who have persistent esophageal eosinophilia despite trial of treatment with a proton pump inhibitor (PPI), with the diagnoses of EoE and gastroesophageal reflux disease (GERD) considered to be mutually exclusive.[1] However new research over the past decade has shown there is an entity in which esophageal eosinophilia responds to high-dose PPI but without a presentation consistent with GERD. This condition has been termed PPI-responsive esophageal eosinophilia (PPI-REE), a new subtype of EoE.[2] Therefore, it has recently been recommended that lack of PPI responsiveness is not part of the diagnostic criteria for EoE.

Because of the complexity of this disease, management remains an ongoing challenge for clinicians. A combination of pharmacotherapy, endoscopic interventions, and dietary restrictions is required, and many patients have experienced incomplete benefit.[3] However, in the past decade, there is promise with the development of new biologic therapies.

Disclosures: Drs H.K. Lehman and W. Lam have no relevant disclosures.
Division of Allergy, Immunology, and Rheumatology, Department of Pediatrics, Jacobs School of Medicine and Biomedical Sciences, University at Buffalo, 1001 Main Street, Buffalo, NY 14203, USA
* Corresponding author.
E-mail address: hkm@buffalo.edu

pediatric.theclinics.com

DEFINITION OF EOSINOPHILIC ESOPHAGITIS

EoE is defined as a clinicopathologic condition that is immune or antigen driven. It is diagnosed with histology, endoscopic appearance, and clinical presentation. It is histologically defined by greater than or equal to 15 eosinophils per high-power field (eos/hpf) along with clinical symptoms of esophageal dysfunction. The definition of EoE is difficult because presenting symptoms are similar to those of GERD. Also, there is the entity of EoE without the presentation of GERD but that responds to PPIs, known has PPI-REE. With emergence of PPI-REE, persistent eosinophilia in the esophagus after 2 months of treatment with a PPI is no longer a criterion for diagnosis of EoE[2] (**Box 1**).

Note that esophageal eosinophilia is not exclusive to EoE.[2] Other diseases in which this occurs include Crohn disease, collagen vascular disease, drug-induced esophagitis, hypereosinophilic syndrome, GERD, and eosinophilic gastroenteritis (see **Box 1**). Because of the nonspecific nature of esophageal eosinophilia, the diagnosis of EoE may be delayed or missed. In a study of 200 adult patients diagnosed with EoE, the median delay in diagnosis was 6 years.[4]

Endoscopic Findings

There are identified endoscopic features that suggest the diagnosis EoE but are not specific and are not included in the criteria for diagnosis. The endoscopic features that were identified in a meta-analysis of 4678 patients with EoE included stacked circular rings, linear furrows, loss of subepithelial vascular pattern, strictures, whitish papules, and small-caliber esophagus.[5]

Histologic Findings

The diagnosis of EoE requires 15 eosinophils/hpf in the esophageal mucosa. Multiple biopsies are required because the diagnosis may be missed with fewer biopsies. In a

---

Box 1
Definition of eosinophilic esophagitis

The diagnostic criteria of EoE include the following:
  Symptoms related to esophageal dysfunction

Peak value of greater than or equal to 15 eosinophils/hpf on esophageal biopsy

Exclusion of differential diagnoses for esophageal eosinophilia

Differential diagnosis of esophageal eosinophilia

GERD

Eosinophilic gastroenteritis

Crohn disease

Connective tissue diseases

Hypereosinophilic syndrome

Infection
  Drug hypersensitivity response

Data from Dellon ES, Liacouras CA, Molina-Infante J, et al. Updated International Consensus Diagnostic Criteria for Eosinophilic Esophagitis: Proceedings of the AGREE Conference. Gastroenterology. 2018;155(4):1022-1033 e1010; and Liacouras CA, Furuta GT, Hirano I, et al. Eosinophilic esophagitis: updated consensus recommendations for children and adults. J Allergy Clin Immunol. 2011;128(1):3-20 e26; quiz 21-22.

study of 102 patients with EoE, the probabilities of the diagnosis with 1, 4, 5, and 6 biopsies of having greater than 15 eosinophils/hpf were 0.63, 0.98, 0.99, and greater than 0.99, respectively.[6]

The pathologic features characteristic of EoE are separated into major and minor features. Major features include intraepithelial eosinophils at a concentration of greater than 15/hpf; eosinophilic microabscesses, which are groups of 4 or more eosinophils within the epithelium; surface layering, where eosinophils aggregate in the surface layers of the epithelium; surface sloughing of squamous cells and eosinophils; and eosinophil degranulation.[7] Minor features include increased basal cell hyperplasia, lengthening of the lamina propria papillae, increased intraepithelial lymphocytes and mast cells, increased intercellular edema, and lamina propria fibrosis.[7]

Laboratory Evaluation

EoE has a strong association with atopy, and laboratory abnormalities associated with atopy are often found in patients with EoE, although they are not part of the diagnostic criteria. Patients with EoE may have slightly increased total immunoglobulin (Ig) E levels, and many patients with EoE have mild peripheral blood eosinophilia,[8,9] with one center finding peripheral eosinophilia a much more common feature of pediatric EoE than adult EoE. A skin testing–based evaluation for specific food allergies and environmental allergies may also be considered in the evaluation of patients with EoE (discussed later).

CLINICAL FEATURES OF EOSINOPHILIC ESOPHAGITIS

Pediatric and adult EoE differ in their clinical presentations. In children, often the first presenting symptoms of EoE are feeding refusal or intolerance, which may be related to the inability of younger children to describe the feeling of dysphagia. Children with EoE also commonly have reflux symptoms, emesis, and abdominal pain. Failure to thrive, chest pain, and diarrhea are other presenting symptoms. Dysphagia and food impaction have been found to be more common in older children and adolescents.[2]

In adults, dysphagia with solid foods and food impaction are the two most commonly reported symptoms. Other symptoms include heartburn, reflux, and chest discomfort. Less commonly than in children, abdominal pain, diarrhea, and weight loss are reported in adult patients with EoE.

On initial history, patients may describe coping strategies that allow them to avoid some of the symptoms of EoE, such as washing down food with liquid, chewing food thoroughly, or avoiding foods that are associated with more dysphagia, such as meats.

Most children and adults with EoE have a personal history of other atopic conditions or a family history of either EoE or atopy.[10]

PATHOGENESIS

The pathogenesis of EoE is driven by various genetic, environmental, and host immune system factors and is not well understood. The presence of increased numbers of eosinophils in the esophageal squamous epithelium is the hallmark of EoE, but increased esophageal eosinophil levels are also present in a multitude of other disorders.[7]

Food and possibly inhaled protein antigens trigger an adaptive T helper type 2 (Th2) cell–mediated response that involves interleukin (IL)-5 and IL-13.[11] IL-5 induces eosinophil growth and an activation factor that activates eosinophils to respond to eotaxin 3, which prolongs their survival. IL-13 also activates eotaxin 3 and calpain 14, known mediators of EoE. Eotaxin 3 gene is induced, which causes an influx of eosinophils into tissue.[7]

Approximately 75% of patients with EoE have evidence of allergy, with most having aeroallergen sensitization and a minority having food allergies.[12] There is evidence for seasonal variability of symptoms and diagnosis of EoE, suggesting these aeroallergen sensitizations are likely a contributing factor.

The complexity of EoE is primarily caused by the mixed picture of IgE-mediated and delayed Th2 responses.[13] In a study by Straumann and colleagues,[14] there were increased levels of eosinophils, T cells, and mast cells in esophageal mucosal biopsies compared with normal levels in stomach and duodenum. There was also increased expression of IL-5 and tumor necrosis factor-alpha in esophageal epithelial biopsy specimens. Also, there are increased levels of systemic and esophageal IgG4 in patients with EoE, suggesting its role in this disease as well.[15] The high levels of IgG4 may play a role in blocking IgE responses and may explain the dissociation between the absence of positive skin tests and effective elimination diets.

EPIDEMIOLOGY

EoE was first described in 1977[16] but it has only been in the last 25 years that the entity became more recognized by gastroenterologists and prevalence data began to be generated. Its estimated prevalence in the United States in an assessment of nationwide commercial insurance claims data from 2009 to 2011 was 56.7 cases per 100,000 persons, with similar rates in both children (50.5 cases per 100,000) and adults (58.9 per 100,000).[17] High prevalence rates have been reported in the United States and Europe, whereas EoE seems to be less common in Asia.[18]

Multiple studies support the perception that the prevalence of EoE has been increasing. It is unclear how much of this increase in prevalence is caused by increased recognition versus increased development of the disease in patients.[19] The annual incidence of new EoE diagnoses increased at the Mayo Clinic and its affiliates from 0.35 cases per 100,000 person-years during 1991 to 1995 to 9.45 cases per 100,000 person-years during 2001 to 2005.[20] A study from a single county in Switzerland found an increase in EoE prevalence from 3.1 cases per 100,000 inhabitants in 1989 to 1991 to 42.8 cases per 100,000 inhabitants in 2007 to 2009.[21] In Denmark, there was a 19.5-fold increase in incidence from 1997 to 2012, in a time during which there was only a 1.9-fold increase in rate of esophageal biopsies performed.[19]

A survey suggested possible variation of prevalence within the United States, with a higher prevalence in northeastern states and lower prevalence in western states.[22] This suggestion was supported by insurance claims–based data, in which United States EoE prevalence by region was most common in the Midwest (71.9 cases per 100,000) and least common in the west (30.9 cases per 100,000).[17]

Overall, male patients are more affected than female patients. Sixteen studies identifying 754 pediatric patients (mean age, 8.6 years) showed that 66% were male.[23] Data from 13 studies evaluating 323 adults (mean age, 38 years) identified that 76% were male.[24] An analysis of insurance claims–based data indicated male predominance as well, with boys accounting for 70.1% of 3933 pediatric cases and for 63.3% of 12,472 adult cases of EoE.[17]

Little is known regarding risk factors for EoE. In a case-control study that included 115 patients with EoE and 225 controls, patients with EoE were significantly less likely to have ever smoked cigarettes or to actively use nonsteroidal antiinflammatory drugs.[25] Early-life exposures considered potential risk factors for EoE include antibiotics use in the first year of life, cesarean delivery, and preterm birth.[26,27]

THE ROLE OF FOOD ALLERGY AND ENVIRONMENTAL ALLERGY IN EOSINOPHILIC ESOPHAGITIS

EoE has been considered a form of food allergy, because avoidance of food proteins in pediatric patients with EoE has been shown to control disease in most, although not all, children with EoE.

In 1995, Kelly and colleagues[28] provided strong evidence that immunologic response to food protein drives EoE. In this study, 10 children with EoE, resistant to standard antireflux medications, were placed on a trial of amino acid–based formula, and symptoms and endoscopic findings were compared before and after this elemental diet. Eight of 10 children experienced complete resolution of their symptoms and the remaining 2 reported significant improvement but not complete resolution. Endoscopic changes included a decrease in maximal esophageal intraepithelial eosinophils from a median of 41/hpf before the formula trial to 0.5/hpf after at least 6 weeks of elemental diet.

Since Kelly and colleagues'[28] initial observation of the effectiveness of an elemental diet, subsequent studies have continued to support its effectiveness in children, and also in adults, with EoE. Liacouras and colleagues[29] presented a large retrospective case series of children with EoE. In this series, 172 patients attempted a completely elemental diet, of which 164 were compliant with the diet. Ninety-seven percent of those able to follow this diet showed significant improvement in esophageal eosinophilia (average 1.1 eos/hpf vs 38.7 eos/hpf before diet) and improved clinical symptoms. A meta-analysis of 13 studies of elemental diet in EoE (12 in children and 1 in adults) found that the overall effectiveness of strict elemental diet in achieving histologic remission of EoE was 90.8% (95% confidence interval, 84.7%–95.5%).[30]

Although food allergy plays an important role in EoE pathogenesis, food allergy testing does not always identify the causative food allergens. Elimination diets based on skin prick testing (SPT) for foods, either alone or in combination with atopy patch testing (APT), result in improvement in some patients with EoE but have much lower efficacy than strictly elemental diets. In 2002, Spergel and colleagues[12] reported on 26 children who underwent elimination diet based on SPT and APT. Following a diet based on avoidance of foods positive on SPT or APT, 18 had complete symptom resolution, 6 had partial improvement, and 2 were lost to follow-up. A recent meta-analysis of 14 studies of allergy testing–directed food elimination for EoE showed an overall 45.5% resolution rate, with a wide 95% confidence interval of 35.4% to 55.7%.[30] Spergel and colleagues[31] have suggested that, because milk is the most common food allergy in patients with EoE and because of the high rate of false-negatives for milk SPT and APT in EoE, a combined empiric milk elimination plus allergy testing–directed elimination of other foods can increase the success rate of directed food elimination to 77%.

In 2006, Kagalwalla and colleagues[32] proposed the concept of an empiric 6-food elimination diet (SFED) to eliminate the food proteins most commonly associated with food allergies and/or EoE. This list included milk, soy, egg, wheat, all nuts, and all seafood. This list was suggested to avoid the limitations of insensitive allergy skin testing in EoE, while still being less restrictive and more palatable than a completely elemental diet. The remission rate with this intervention (defined as <10 eos/hpf on esophageal biopsy) was 74%. Follow-up studies by the same group retrospectively evaluated single-food reintroductions to identify the specific foods responsible for EoE disorder.[33] Children who achieved histologic remission after initial SFED sequentially reintroduced the excluded foods. If remission was maintained after a food reintroduction, then that food was retained in the diet. If there was an EoE exacerbation with a given food, then it was eliminated. Endoscopy was performed at least 6 weeks from the time each new food was reintroduced. This reintroduction process revealed that a single offending food was the cause of inflammation in 72% of these children, 2 foods were allergens in 8%, and 3 foods were causative in 8%. Eleven percent of patients tolerated reintroduction of all 6 foods without recurrence of their esophagitis. Subsequent studies in adults have shown similar results for the efficacy of SFED and successive reintroductions.[30]

Multiple studies show that milk tends to be the most commonly identified trigger in EoE, with wheat, egg, and soy/legumes being other frequent culprits. Given the minor role of nut and seafood allergies in EoE, a modified 4-food elimination diet (FFED) has been proposed and studied. Molina-Infante and colleagues[34] showed that 54% of adult patients responded to an FFED diet eliminating dairy, egg, wheat, and legumes. In this same group, 72% of adults responded when an SFED was used as rescue therapy for those that did not respond to FFED. Kagalwalla and colleagues[35] found the FFED to be effective in inducing remission in 62% of a population with pediatric EoE.

Besides foods, there is also evidence that aeroallergen sensitization may act as a contributor to EoE. Many patients with EoE also have allergic asthma and/or allergic rhinitis and are sensitized to environmental inhalant allergens. There is evidence that EoE symptoms worsen in some patients during the spring and/or fall pollen seasons.[28,36] In addition, a single-center retrospective study showed that time of initial EoE symptoms was correlated with times of peak grass pollen and ragweed pollen counts at local pollen counting stations.[37]

A study by Sugnanam and colleagues[38] evaluating food and aeroallergen sensitizations in children with EoE showed that younger patients with EoE showed more IgE and patch test sensitization to foods, whereas older children showed greater IgE sensitization to inhalant allergens. However, the causative nature of these positive tests was not explored in this study.

It has recently been noted that a small but significant subset of patients with EoE who have failed SFED are sensitized to fresh fruits and vegetables, suggesting an oral allergy syndrome–like cross-reactivity with plant allergens, such as profilins and birch pollen.[31]

TREATMENT OF EOSINOPHILIC ESOPHAGITIS
Conventional Pharmacologic Therapies

For treatment of EoE, topical steroids (ie, swallowed fluticasone or budesonide) achieve successful remission in up to 80% of patients, although 10% of patients are refractory to this treatment, and, when steroids are discontinued in patients once controlled, disease nearly always recurs. Although no topical steroid formulations are approved specifically for EoE, recommended dosing of fluticasone from consensus guidelines (swallowed through a metered-dose inhaler) is 440 to 880 mg twice daily for adults or 88 to 440 mg twice to 4 times daily (to a maximal daily adult dose) for children. Recommended dosing of budesonide (swallowed as a viscous suspension) is 1 mg daily for children less than 10 years old or 2 mg daily for older children and adults.[3]

Prednisone may be useful if topical steroids are not effective.[39] However, it is recommended that systemic steroids be used only in emergency cases, such as to treat severe dysphagia and weight loss, or for treatment during hospitalization. Because of the potential for significant side effects and the availability of other treatments that are effective in most cases, the long-term use of systemic steroids is not recommended for EoE.[3]

The role of PPI therapy in treatment of EoE has evolved over time. Originally, the diagnosis of EoE was dependent on a failure of PPIs to resolve symptoms related to esophageal dysfunction. The role of PPI treatment failure in the diagnosis of EoE was readdressed at the AGREE (A Working Group on PPI-REE) conference in 2017 involving experts from 14 countries.[2] It was concluded that there is significant overlap between PPI-REE and EoE, and that GERD and EoE are not mutually exclusive.

Dietary Interventions

The 3 main approaches in dietary management are (1) a strictly elemental (amino acid) formula-based diet; (2) empiric food elimination, based on most common allergic triggers (ie, milk, wheat, egg, soy, nuts, and seafood); and (3) allergy test–directed elimination, based on positive allergy skin prick test and/or patch test results.

Each dietary approach offers different pros and cons for patients with EoE (**Table 1**). Although elemental diets with amino acid–based formulas are highly effective, they are unpalatable and are better tolerated by infants than by older children with EoE. The frequent need for nasogastric tube or gastrostomy placement and the high cost of elemental formula are also negatives of the strict elemental diet. In general, elemental diet is mainly an option for treating EoE in children with multiple food allergies, failure to thrive, and severe disease in which a strict diet with multiple eliminations is ineffective. Directed elimination diets, based on skin test and/or atopy patch test results, offers better long-term tolerability for most patients. Skin tests and patch tests have variable sensitivity and specificity for different food triggers, and atopy patch tests are not standardized. Ability of testing-directed elimination diets to achieve histologic remission of EoE was estimated at only 45.5% in a meta-analysis,[30] but recently a modified approach of elimination guided by SPT and APT combined with empiric milk elimination has been suggested to achieve a response rate of 77%.[31]

Empiric elimination diets, in the form of SFED or FFED, have good efficacy, are more tolerable for many patients compared with elemental diet, and avoid the need for gastrostomy-tube placement. However, with the elimination of 4 or 6 major food categories (dairy, egg, legumes, wheat, and in the case of SFED also nuts and seafood), achieving appropriate nutrition is still challenging and requires the involvement of an experienced nutritionist.

Molina-Infante and colleagues[40] have evaluated the effectiveness of a step-up empiric dietary strategy in pediatric and adult patients with EoE, as an alternative to a

Table 1
Comparison of dietary therapies for eosinophilic esophagitis

Diet	Pros	Cons
Elemental formula	Effective in nearly all patients	High cost Requires NG or PEG tube in most patients Decreased QOL Negative psychosocial impacts
Six food elimination	Effective in many patients Some foods may be able to be reintroduced	Moderately high cost Potential nutritional deficits Serial EGD may be needed to assess response to food removal and reintroductions
Guided elimination	Often requires fewer food avoidances (depends on number of positive tests)	Extensive allergy testing required Less effective in many studies than other interventions Nutritional deficits may occur if many foods are removed

Abbreviations: EGD, esophagogastroduodenoscopy; NG, nasogastric; PEG, percutaneous endoscopic gastrostomy; QOL, quality of life.

traditional SFED. Patients with EoE unresponsive to PPI therapy underwent a 2-food elimination diet (milk and gluten-containing grains). Nonresponders were offered an FFED (2-food elimination diet plus elimination of egg and legumes) and subsequent nonresponders were placed onto a 6-food-group elimination diet (FFED plus withdrawal of nuts and seafood). Remission was achieved in 43%, 60%, and 79% of patients with the 2-food elimination diet, FFED, and SFED, respectively.

Food reintroduction is a key aspect of the long-term management of EoE. Following remission with any of the major dietary interventions, foods should be gradually reintroduced, with observation for recurrence of symptoms of EoE and consideration of serial repeat endoscopies. Spergel and Shuker[41] suggest reintroducing the least allergic foods first, such as fruits and vegetables, whereas the most allergenic foods (milk, egg, wheat, and soy) are left to last.

Esophageal Dilation

For symptomatic patients with strictures, esophageal dilation is an option if medical or dietary therapy have failed, but it does not address the underlying inflammation in EoE. Because of the low rate of esophageal strictures in children with EoE, most esophageal dilations have been performed in adult patients with EoE. Early reports of outcomes of esophageal dilation for EoE suggested high complication rates, with 5% of patients experiencing esophageal perforation and 7% requiring hospitalization for chest pain.[42] However, more recent data suggest that the rate of perforation is much lower. A 2017 meta-analysis of 37 studies found that perforation and postprocedure hospitalization occurred in only 0.03% of dilations for EoE.[43]

Biologics

Anti–IL-5 monoclonal antibodies and other biologics targeting Th2 inflammation seem promising as therapy for EoE because of their low side effect profile but, to date, none have become US Food and Drug Administration approved for treatment of EoE. Anti–IL-5 therapies were some of the first to be investigated for use in EoE. These products were chosen because IL-5 is a key cytokine critical for survival of eosinophils. A trial of reslizumab, an anti–IL-5 humanized monoclonal antibody, in pediatric patients with EoE showed significant decrease compared with placebo in peak eosinophil count per high-power field on esophageal biopsy (but counts were still above the levels consist with histologic remission) and there was no significant difference of Physician Global Assessment scores compared with placebo.[44] Two trials of another anti–IL-5 monoclonal antibody, mepolizumab, in EoE failed to reach their primary outcome measures of significant histologic remission rate (reduction of esophageal eosinophils to <5/hpf).[45,46]

Recent trials of biologics directed at IL-13 and at the IL-4Rα subunit (a component of both the IL-4 and IL-13 receptors) have shown significant reductions in esophageal eosinophilia and improvement in symptoms of EoE. A phase II, randomized, double-blind, placebo-controlled, parallel-group clinical trial was undertaken to evaluate the efficacy and safety of RPC4046, an anti–IL-13 monoclonal antibody in adult subjects with EoE.[47] Significant improvement from placebo was seen in eosinophil count per high-power field on esophageal biopsy, as well as EoE endoscopic reference score and the clinician's global assessment of disease severity score.

A double-blinded, randomized, placebo-controlled, phase II trial was recently completed to evaluate long-term safety and clinical efficacy of dupilumab, a monoclonal antibody against IL-4Rα, for use in EoE. Initial positive results of this study have been presented in abstract form but are not yet published.[48]

The outcomes of these recent trials of biologics targeting IL-4 and/or IL-13 seem more promising than those reported in previous trials of biologics targeting IL-5, but the ultimate success of these therapies remain to be determined in upcoming phase III trials. In addition, in several trials to date, it seems that outcomes improve when conventional therapy, such as PPIs or topical steroids, was given in conjunction with a biologic.

SUMMARY

EoE is a newly defined condition that has dramatically increased in prevalence in the last several decades. It may occur at any age, but the clinical presentation in young children is often more vague than the classic solid food dysphagia and food impacting that are the major presenting symptoms of EoE in adults and adolescents. Successful therapies exist, including medications and dietary modifications, but disease typically recurs when the successful intervention is discontinued. Although no biologic therapies are currently approved for the treatment of EoE, clinical trials are ongoing and these therapies that specifically target aspects of Th2-mediated inflammation may play a role in the treatment of EoE in the future.

REFERENCES

1. Furuta GT, Liacouras CA, Collins MH, et al. Eosinophilic esophagitis in children and adults: a systematic review and consensus recommendations for diagnosis and treatment. Gastroenterology 2007;133(4):1342–63.
2. Dellon ES, Liacouras CA, Molina-Infante J, et al. Updated international consensus diagnostic criteria for eosinophilic esophagitis: proceedings of the AGREE conference. Gastroenterology 2018;155(4):1022–33.e10.
3. Liacouras CA, Furuta GT, Hirano I, et al. Eosinophilic esophagitis: updated consensus recommendations for children and adults. J Allergy Clin Immunol 2011;128(1):3–20.e26 [quiz: 21–2].
4. Schoepfer AM, Safroneeva E, Bussmann C, et al. Delay in diagnosis of eosinophilic esophagitis increases risk for stricture formation in a time-dependent manner. Gastroenterology 2013;145(6):1230–6.e1–2.
5. Kim HP, Vance RB, Shaheen NJ, et al. The prevalence and diagnostic utility of endoscopic features of eosinophilic esophagitis: a meta-analysis. Clin Gastroenterol Hepatol 2012;10(9):988–96.e5.
6. Nielsen JA, Lager DJ, Lewin M, et al. The optimal number of biopsy fragments to establish a morphologic diagnosis of eosinophilic esophagitis. Am J Gastroenterol 2014;109(4):515.
7. Hogan SP, Mishra A, Brandt EB, et al. A critical role for eotaxin in experimental oral antigen-induced eosinophilic gastrointestinal allergy. Proc Natl Acad Sci U S A 2000;97(12):6681–6.
8. Erwin EA, James HR, Gutekunst HM, et al. Serum IgE measurement and detection of food allergy in pediatric patients with eosinophilic esophagitis. Ann Allergy Asthma Immunol 2010;104(6):496–502.
9. Dellon ES, Gibbs WB, Fritchie KJ, et al. Clinical, endoscopic, and histologic findings distinguish eosinophilic esophagitis from gastroesophageal reflux disease. Clin Gastroenterol Hepatol 2009;7(12):1305–13.
10. Noel RJ, Putnam PE, Rothenberg ME. Eosinophilic esophagitis. N Engl J Med 2004;351(9):940–1.
11. Mishra A, Hogan SP, Lee JJ, et al. Fundamental signals that regulate eosinophil homing to the gastrointestinal tract. J Clin Invest 1999;103(12):1719–27.
12. Spergel JM, Beausoleil JL, Mascarenhas M, et al. The use of skin prick tests and patch tests to identify causative foods in eosinophilic esophagitis. J Allergy Clin Immunol 2002;109(2):363–8.

13. Rothenberg ME. Eosinophilic gastrointestinal disorders (EGID). J Allergy Clin Immunol 2004;113(1):11–28 [quiz: 29].

14. Straumann A, Bauer M, Fischer B, et al. Idiopathic eosinophilic esophagitis is associated with a T(H)2-type allergic inflammatory response. J Allergy Clin Immunol 2001;108(6):954–61.

15. Wright BL, Kulis M, Guo R, et al. Food-specific IgG4 is associated with eosinophilic esophagitis. J Allergy Clin Immunol 2016;138(4):1190–2.e3.

16. Dobbins JW, Sheahan DG, Behar J. Eosinophilic gastroenteritis with esophageal involvement. Gastroenterology 1977;72(6):1312–6.

17. Dellon ES, Jensen ET, Martin CF, et al. Prevalence of eosinophilic esophagitis in the United States. Clin Gastroenterol Hepatol 2014;12(4):589–96.e1.

18. Kinoshita Y, Ishimura N, Oshima N, et al. Systematic review: eosinophilic esophagitis in Asian countries. World J Gastroenterol 2015;21(27):8433–40.

19. Dellon ES, Erichsen R, Baron JA, et al. The increasing incidence and prevalence of eosinophilic oesophagitis outpaces changes in endoscopic and biopsy practice: national population-based estimates from Denmark. Aliment Pharmacol Ther 2015;41(7):662–70.

20. Prasad GA, Alexander JA, Schleck CD, et al. Epidemiology of eosinophilic esophagitis over three decades in Olmsted County, Minnesota. Clin Gastroenterol Hepatol 2009;7(10):1055–61.

21. Hruz P, Straumann A, Bussmann C, et al. Escalating incidence of eosinophilic esophagitis: a 20-year prospective, population-based study in Olten County, Switzerland. J Allergy Clin Immunol 2011;128(6):1349–50.e5.

22. Spergel JM, Book WM, Mays E, et al. Variation in prevalence, diagnostic criteria, and initial management options for eosinophilic gastrointestinal diseases in the United States. J Pediatr Gastroenterol Nutr 2011;52(3):300–6.

23. Walsh SV, Antonioli DA, Goldman H, et al. Allergic esophagitis in children: a clinicopathological entity. Am J Surg Pathol 1999;23(4):390–6.

24. Zimmerman SL, Levine MS, Rubesin SE, et al. Idiopathic eosinophilic esophagitis in adults: the ringed esophagus. Radiology 2005;236(1):159–65.

25. Koutlas NT, Eluri S, Rusin S, et al. Impact of smoking, alcohol consumption, and NSAID use on risk for and phenotypes of eosinophilic esophagitis. Dis Esophagus 2018;31(1):1–7.

26. Jensen ET, Bertelsen RJ. Assessing early life factors for eosinophilic esophagitis: lessons from other allergic diseases. Curr Treat Options Gastroenterol 2016;14(1):39–50.

27. Jensen ET, Kappelman MD, Kim HP, et al. Early life exposures as risk factors for pediatric eosinophilic esophagitis. J Pediatr Gastroenterol Nutr 2013;57(1):67–71.

28. Kelly KJ, Lazenby AJ, Rowe PC, et al. Eosinophilic esophagitis attributed to gastroesophageal reflux: improvement with an amino acid-based formula. Gastroenterology 1995;109(5):1503–12.

29. Liacouras CA, Spergel JM, Ruchelli E, et al. Eosinophilic esophagitis: a 10-year experience in 381 children. Clin Gastroenterol Hepatol 2005;3(12):1198–206.

30. Arias A, Gonzalez-Cervera J, Tenias JM, et al. Efficacy of dietary interventions for inducing histologic remission in patients with eosinophilic esophagitis: a systematic review and meta-analysis. Gastroenterology 2014;146(7):1639–48.

31. Spergel JM, Brown-Whitehorn TF, Cianferoni A, et al. Identification of causative foods in children with eosinophilic esophagitis treated with an elimination diet. J Allergy Clin Immunol 2012;130(2):461–7.e5.

32. Kagalwalla AF, Sentongo TA, Ritz S, et al. Effect of six-food elimination diet on clinical and histologic outcomes in eosinophilic esophagitis. Clin Gastroenterol Hepatol 2006;4(9):1097–102.

33. Kagalwalla AF, Shah A, Li BU, et al. Identification of specific foods responsible for inflammation in children with eosinophilic esophagitis successfully treated with empiric elimination diet. J Pediatr Gastroenterol Nutr 2011;53(2):145–9.

34. Molina-Infante J, Arias A, Barrio J, et al. Four-food group elimination diet for adult eosinophilic esophagitis: a prospective multicenter study. J Allergy Clin Immunol 2014;134(5):1093–9.e1.

35. Kagalwalla AF, Wechsler JB, Amsden K, et al. Efficacy of a 4-food elimination diet for children with eosinophilic esophagitis. Clin Gastroenterol Hepatol 2017; 15(11):1698–707.e7.

36. Ram G, Lee J, Ott M, et al. Seasonal exacerbation of esophageal eosinophilia in children with eosinophilic esophagitis and allergic rhinitis. Ann Allergy Asthma Immunol 2015;115(3):224–8.e1.

37. Fahey L, Robinson G, Weinberger K, et al. Correlation between aeroallergen levels and new diagnosis of eosinophilic esophagitis in New York City. J Pediatr Gastroenterol Nutr 2017;64(1):22–5.

38. Sugnanam KK, Collins JT, Smith PK, et al. Dichotomy of food and inhalant allergen sensitization in eosinophilic esophagitis. Allergy 2007;62(11):1257–60.

39. Dellon ES, Gonsalves N, Hirano I, et al. ACG clinical guideline: evidenced based approach to the diagnosis and management of esophageal eosinophilia and eosinophilic esophagitis (EoE). Am J Gastroenterol 2013;108(5):679–92 [quiz: 693].

40. Molina-Infante J, Arias A, Alcedo J, et al. Step-up empiric elimination diet for pediatric and adult eosinophilic esophagitis: the 2-4-6 study. J Allergy Clin Immunol 2018;141(4):1365–72.

41. Spergel JM, Shuker M. Nutritional management of eosinophilic esophagitis. Gastrointest Endosc Clin N Am 2008;18(1):179–94, xi.

42. Hirano I. Dilation in eosinophilic esophagitis: to do or not to do? Gastrointest Endosc 2010;71(4):713–4.

43. Dougherty M, Runge TM, Eluri S, et al. Esophageal dilation with either bougie or balloon technique as a treatment for eosinophilic esophagitis: a systematic review and meta-analysis. Gastrointest Endosc 2017;86(4):581–91.e3.

44. Spergel JM, Rothenberg ME, Collins MH, et al. Reslizumab in children and adolescents with eosinophilic esophagitis: results of a double-blind, randomized, placebo-controlled trial. J Allergy Clin Immunol 2012;129(2):456–63, 463.e1-3.

45. Straumann A, Conus S, Grzonka P, et al. Anti-interleukin-5 antibody treatment (mepolizumab) in active eosinophilic oesophagitis: a randomised, placebo-controlled, double-blind trial. Gut 2010;59(1):21–30.

46. Assa'ad AH, Gupta SK, Collins MH, et al. An antibody against IL-5 reduces numbers of esophageal intraepithelial eosinophils in children with eosinophilic esophagitis. Gastroenterology 2011;141(5):1593–604.

47. Hirano I, Collins MH, Assouline-Dayan Y, et al. RPC4046, a monoclonal antibody against IL13, reduces histologic and endoscopic activity in patients with eosinophilic esophagitis. Gastroenterology 2018;156(3):592–603.e10.

48. Hirano I, Dellon E, Hamilton J, et al. Dupilumab efficacy and safety in adult patients with active eosinophilic esophagitis: a randomized, double blind, placebo controlled phase 2 trial. World Congress of Gastroenterology at ACG. Orlando, October 15-18, 2017.

Pediatric Inner-City Asthma

Divya Seth, MD[a],*, Shweta Saini, MD[b], Pavadee Poowuttikul, MD[c]

KEYWORDS

- Asthma • Inner city • Children • Asthma research networks

KEY POINTS

- Inner-city asthma is often severe and is associated with increased morbidity and mortality.
- Multiple factors contribute significantly to the disease burden, including biological factors, environmental factors, care access, and socioeconomic hardship.
- Risk factors concentrated in these areas such as environmental allergens (cockroach and mouse) and pollutants contribute to increased morbidity.
- Remedial measures focused on reduced exposures to these allergens as well as tobacco smoke, omalizumab, and immunotherapy have been shown to be helpful in control of symptoms in this population.

INTRODUCTION

Inner cities are defined as poor and large urban/metropolitan areas where at least 20% of the households have incomes below the federal poverty level.[1] Several risk factors related to poverty and urban environment independently contribute to increase in asthma morbidity in these children and their daily lifestyle.[1] Although these factors may not be the only causes of asthma development in the children in the inner city, it is certain that many of them contribute to its severity. These risk factors related to poverty and urban environments will be discussed in this article.

PREVALENCE

Asthma is among the most common chronic diseases, affecting over 9.5% of children in the United States.[2] The prevalence of childhood asthma has increased over the last decade and appears to be higher in inner-city children (12.9%) versus noninner-city children (10.6%).[3] Ethnic minority children also have much higher prevalence of asthma (African American 17.1%, Puerto Rican 19.8%, and Caucasian 9.6%).[3]

Conflict of Interest: The authors declare no relevant conflict of interest.
[a] Division of Allergy/Immunology, Department of Pediatrics, Children's Hospital of Michigan, Wayne State University School of Medicine, 3950 Beaubien, 4th Floor, Pediatric Specialty Building, Detroit, MI 48201, USA; [b] Division of Hospital Medicine, Department of Pediatrics, Children's Hospital of Michigan, Wayne State University School of Medicine, Detroit, MI, USA; [c] Division of Allergy/Immunology, Department of Pediatrics, Children's Hospital of Michigan, Wayne State University School of Medicine, Detroit, MI, USA
* Corresponding author.
E-mail address: dseth@dmc.org

MORBIDITY AND MORTALITY

In general, pediatric asthma morbidity is measured by asthma symptoms, activity limitation, asthma exacerbations, and the effect of the disease on the caregiver.[1] Although the prevalence of asthma exacerbations decreased from 61.7% in 2001 to 53.7% in 2016,[4] up to 16.7% of children with asthma still had an asthma exacerbation that required an emergency department (ED) or an urgent care (UC) visit in 2016. In spite of the fact that death related to asthma should be preventable, the mortality rate for children with asthma is at 2.8 cases per million population per year.[5]

It is possible that inner-city children with asthma have more severe disease, needing more medication to control their asthma than noninner-city children. It is hypothesized that decreased responsiveness to corticosteroids can be an underlying cause of this difficult-to- control asthma; however, this hypothesis needs to be further investigated.[6]

Many risk factors related to poverty and urban environment adversely impact asthma severity in inner-city children. These risk factors include increase in certain allergens (mouse and cockroach) sensitization/exposure, environmental tobacco smoke (ETS) exposure, vitamin D insufficiency/deficiency, stress, and obesity. Out of these risk factors, allergen and ETS exposure are noted to be the most important risk factors of severe asthma in the inner-city population.[7]

In the last 15 years, the National Institutes of Allergy and Infectious Diseases (NIAID) funded major research networks to improve asthma care for inner-city children. Three important inner-city asthma networks are the National Cooperative Inner-City Asthma Study (NCICAS), the Inner City Asthma Study (ICAS), and the Inner City Asthma Consortium (ICAC).[6] The results from the NCICAS confirmed that lack of access to health care, poor adherence to asthma medications, childhood behavioral problems, and allergen sensitization are important risk factors contributing to increased asthma morbidity in inner-city children.[6,8]

The next section will describe the effects of the individual risk factors on inner-city asthma in detail.

RISK FACTORS FOR INNER-CITY ASTHMA
Allergen Exposure and Sensitization

Exposure to household pests such as cockroach and mice is much higher in inner-city areas, which contributes to poor asthma control. Cockroach (36.8%), house dust mite (34.9%), and cat dander (22.7%) are the main allergens implicated in sensitization for children with inner-city asthma.[9] Mold is also a factor in poor asthma control. Exposure to these allergens must be curtailed in order to achieve asthma control.

Cockroach

Inner-city areas have high rates of cockroach infestation.[10–12] Sensitization and exposure to cockroach can contribute to increased asthma morbidity including ED visits and hospitalizations.[9] Home interventions to reduce exposure to cockroaches, including extermination, resulted in a significant decrease in asthma morbidity.[13,14]

Mold

Mold exposure has been associated with increased asthma morbidity and mortality,[15] particularly *Alternaria,* which has been associated with increased asthma hospitalizations.[16] Houses with increased dampness and cat and cockroach infestation have high mold levels.[17] Inner-city schools have high levels of *Aspergillus, Cladosporium,* and *Penicillium* molds,[18] which can contribute to increased symptoms. Reduction in mold exposure significantly decreased asthma symptoms as well as exacerbations in inner-city children.[19]

Dust Mites

Inner-city homes have high levels of dust mite allergens, particularly in the bed-rooms.[20–22] While there is no clear association between dust mite exposure and asthma morbidity, some studies have shown that dust mite sensitization is associated with frequent symptoms and increased use of rescue medications.[9,16,23,24]

Reduction of house dust mite allergen levels has been shown to have a beneficial effect on asthma control and improved morbidity, specifically, patients experienced fewer hospitalizations and office visits for asthma and fewer days with symptoms.[14]

Mouse

Inner-city homes, particularly in northeastern and midwestern US cities, have high levels of mouse allergens, with highest levels in the kitchen.[25] Mouse and cockroach infestation are often found to coexist.[26] Mouse allergen exposure was associated with wheezing during infancy[27] and wheezing and atopy later in childhood.[28,29] Studies conducted in Baltimore, Maryland, found that mouse allergen exposure was more closely associated with asthma morbidity compared with other indoor allergens.[30,31]

Inner-city schools have also been shown to have high levels of mouse allergens,[32,33] which contributes to missed school days caused by asthma.[33]

Reduction of mouse allergen levels in ICAS resulted in less sleep disruption, care-taker burden, and missed school but did not reduce asthma symptoms or medical utilization.[34]

Cat and Dog

High levels of pet allergens are present in homes with a cat or dog.[35] Studies have shown variable results regarding the effect of pet allergens on development of asthma or atopic disease. Some studies showed that cat and dog exposure may prevent development of asthma[36] and allergen sensitization.[37,38] Other studies concluded that pet exposure led to higher rates of dog sensitization[39] and development of asthma and eczema.[40] Exposure to high levels of cat allergens in homes of sensitized children resulted in higher asthma severity,[41] frequent wheezing and rescue medica-tion use,[42] asthma exacerbation,[43] and hospitalization.[44] On the other hand, NCICAS did not show any association between cat allergen exposure and asthma morbidity.[9]

Environmental intervention in a study reduced both cat and dog allergens; however, there was no significant decrease in medication use, asthma symptoms, or exacerba-tion.[45] In the ICAS, the environmental interventions significantly decreased cat allergen levels but not dog allergen.[14] The authors did not notice any significant asso-ciation between cat allergen reduction and asthma morbidity.[14]

Infections

Certain infections are noted to be important triggers of asthma. These particular infec-tious agents include rhinovirus and endotoxin, and their effects on asthma have been studied extensively.

Children younger than 5 years old with rhinovirus-induced acute respiratory illness are more likely to be diagnosed with asthma compared to respiratory illnesses from other viruses.[46] Rhinovirus is also a well-known trigger for asthma exacerbation. Also, rhinovirus infection in early childhood can increase the risk of asthma develop-ment.[47] The results from the Childhood Origins of Asthma (COAST) study[47] showed that rhinovirus infection was related to wheezing during the first 3 years of life and the loss of pulmonary function in early school years. This relation was not seen in children who had respiratory syncytial virus (RSV) induced wheezing.

Airborne endotoxin exposure is another risk factor of wheezing and asthma.[10,48,49] Endotoxin is part of the outer membrane lipopolysaccharide of gram-negative bacteria. Exposure to moisture sources and organic waste, commonly seen in inner-city areas, is associated with endotoxin exposure.[48] Inner-city schools have been shown to have high endotoxin concentrations,[49] more so than the inner-city homes. Exposure to high levels of airborne endotoxin at school is associated with increased asthma symptoms in nonatopic asthmatic children.[50]

Seasonal Variations

Inner-city children with asthma typically have more frequent asthma exacerbations during the fall-winter months rather than the summer months.[51] This seasonal variation in asthma exacerbation appears to be related to an allergen-induced immunoglobulin E (IgE)-mediated mechanism. In the Inner City Anti-IgE therapy for Asthma (ICATA) study, asthma exacerbations in inner-city children and young adults during the fall season were almost fully suppressed by the use of anti-IgE monoclonal antibody (omalizumab) therapy in addition to conventional asthma treatment.[52] Similar findings were reported in the Preventative Omalizumab or Step-up therapy for Fall Exacerbations (PROSE) study, where significant reduction in fall asthma exacerbations were achieved after omalizumab therapy 4 to 6 weeks prior to the return to school.[53]

Pollution

Air pollution leads to an increase in asthma symptoms and decreased lung function and potentially contributes to asthma development.[54,55] Inner-city areas are known to be affected by sources of air pollution, particularly traffic and power generation.[54] Nitrogen dioxide, particulate matter, ozone, sulfur dioxide, carbon monoxide, and lead are common outdoor pollutants.[56] Indoor air pollution, in the forms of particulate matter, nitrogen dioxide, and ozone, can be further created by the penetration of outdoor pollutants to indoor environment.[57]

Activities like smoking, cooking, and cleaning, and heating/cooling systems can produce indoor air pollutants.[57,58] As previously mentioned, ETS exposure has been noted to be the single most important risk factors of severe asthma in the inner-city population.[7,8,57] Besides its adverse effects on asthma, ETS is also a well-known cause of asthma development[59,60] and a trigger of asthma exacerbation.[61] Prenatal and postnatal passive ETS exposure can increase the risk of wheezing and asthma by 20%.[59] The risk of asthma at the age of 7 correlates with prenatal ETS exposure.[60] Furthermore, asthmatic children exposed to ETS have more asthma symptoms and ED visits and are twice as likely to be admitted to the hospital.[61]

Thirdhand smoke is residual tobacco-related gases and chemicals that are present on indoor surfaces, including carpets, furniture, blankets, or toys, from which they are released into the air after the secondhand smoke is released in the air.[62] Although the asthma risks of thirdhand smoke exposure are less well described, evidence has shown that it is likely to adversely affect asthma symptoms as well as the secondhand smoke exposure.[62]

Poor indoor air quality in inner-city homes may also be related to poor ventilation.[58,63] In a study by Hansel and colleagues,[64] use of a gas stove, stove/oven, and space heater caused an increase in indoor nitrogen dioxide levels, which contributed to increased asthma symptoms.

Nonadherence to Medication

Medication adherence, proper inhaler technique, and avoidance of triggers have been identified as key factors for asthma control. A study was conducted to identify the risk factors for poor medication adherence and thus asthma morbidity in inner-city children. These included concerns about medication adverse effects, multiple caregivers, trouble with obtaining appointments, nonavailablity of medication in the house when needed, and child refusing to take medication.[65]

The Asthma Control Evaluation (ACE) study further emphasized the importance of medication adherence in control of asthma.[66] The study showed that in inner-city children, guideline-based asthma care and strict medication adherence can help to achieve asthma control.

A study in Detroit showed that the most severe asthmatics were more likely to miss medications due to running out even when refills are available. The majority of asthmatic children who were hospitalized reported lack of medical supplies and prescription medications in the home.[67]

Family–physician partnership geared at communication, trust, and respect has helped to increase medication adherence in these families.[68]

Stress, Psychological Issues, and Depression

Poor asthma control in inner-city children is associated with caregiver stress. Multiple studies have shown that maternal depression and stress in the initial 3 years of life increase risk of recurrent wheezing at 3 years and asthma at age 7 in children.[60,69,70] Wing and colleagues[71] conducted a study and found domestic violence to be associated with lifetime asthma in inner-city children.

Vitamin D Deficiency

Vitamin D deficiency has been speculated to play a role in the development of asthma.[72,73] Prenatal vitamin D supplementation may be protective against recurrent wheezing early in the infant's life.[74] Liu and colleagues,[7] however, did not find any significant effect of vitamin D on asthma severity in inner-city children.

Obesity

Obesity has been associated with increased asthma symptoms and exacerbations irrespective of allergic sensitization.[75–77] Lung function and asthma control improved in obese children after weight loss.[78] Liu and colleagues,[7] however, did not notice any significant effect of obesity on asthma severity.

Immune Dysregulation

Immune system dysregulation can increase risk of allergic sensitization and asthma. This can occur prenatally, at birth, or during infancy.[1,79] Under ICAC (2002), the Urban Environment and Childhood Asthma (URECA, 2004) study was initiated with the aim of determining immunologic causes of asthma in inner-city children.[80] As part of URECA, a birth cohort of inner-city newborns at risk for asthma has been followed to identify prenatal exposures and maternal factors that can affect development of newborn immune system and cytokine responses.[81–83] Results from the study so far have identified certain environmental factors such as ethnicity, birth weight/gestational age, season of birth, and maternal asthma/use of inhaled corticosteroids that can affect newborn immune responses.[79]

Epigenetics

Various genes have been identified as affecting asthma.[84] Epigenetics is a science that aims to study the effect of environmental exposures in causing functional changes such as methylation of selective genes that are relevant to asthma, particularly for inner-city children. Nasal epithelia in inner-city children with persistent asthma has been shown to have differential methylation patterns (DMRs).[85] There were significant differences in methylation between asthmatic children and nonasthmatic controls. Of these, 48 DMRs were associated with tobacco smoke.[85]

INTERVENTIONS FOR INNER-CITY ASTHMA
Family-Based Interventions

As multiple risk factors contribute to high asthma morbidity in the inner-city population, asthma management and interventions for this high-risk group are frequently challenging.[8] As mentioned previously, factors associated with poverty including socioeconomic hardship and lack of knowledge or participation in the health care system contribute to high asthma morbidity in inner-city children. The major NIAID-funded network, NCICAS, focused on family-based interventions. The results from the NCICAS identified that family-based interventions including partnering the family with asthma-trained social workers can reduce asthma-related morbidity by helping families access better medical care.[13] Furthermore, the results from ACE study (part of the ICAC) also revealed that inner-city asthma children can achieve good asthma control with optimal medication adherence to proper asthma treatment.[66]

Anti-immunoglobulin E Monoclonal Antibody Therapy

As previously discussed, allergen sensitization/exposure is a major risk factor of inner-city asthma that leads to asthma exacerbations despite the use of aggressive inhaled corticosteroid treatment. This fact has been confirmed by both the ICATA[52] and PROSE[53] studies. In both studies, anti-IgE monoclonal antibody (omalizumab) can significantly reduce asthma exacerbations and reduce the dose of inhaled corticosteroid therapy compared with placebo. Omalizumab is able to reduce fall and spring asthma exacerbations, with maximal benefit seen in those who had recent asthma exacerbations.[52]

Other than reducing seasonal asthma exacerbations, omalizumab appears to be able to alter the immune response to rhinovirus also.[86,87] Children who received omalizumab demonstrated increased interferon alpha (IFN-α) against rhinovirus.[87] The results from PROSE study revealed that omalizumab can decrease frequency and duration of rhinovirus infection and also reduce peak rhinovirus shedding.[86]

Immunotherapy

As allergen sensitization and exposure play important roles in inner-city asthma morbidity, allergen immunotherapy (IT) potentially can be beneficial to inner-city asthma patients.[8] It is known that IT is a disease-modifying therapy with sustained benefits, unlike other pharmacologic treatments for asthma.[88] As mentioned concerning the risk factors of inner-city asthma, cockroach allergy and exposure are associated with higher asthma morbidity in inner-city children. The ICAC study evaluated the clinical effects of cockroach IT along with biomarkers, such as cockroach IgE or cockroach IgG4 levels, which link to clinical outcome of the IT in inner-city patients with asthma.[89]

The important findings from the ICAC study regarding cockroach IT are that significant but inconsistent changes in serum-specific cockroach IgE levels were identified after German cockroach sublingual immunotherapy (SLIT). In contrast, use of cockroach subcutaneous immunotherapy (SCIT) resulted in significant and substantial immunologic changes in the treatment group. These results conclude that SCIT might be a better option for cockroach IT in inner-city patients with asthma.[89]

Environmental Interventions

Population-level environmental interventions such as prohibiting smoking in public places, vehicle emission regulations, and replacing indoor gas heaters in schools with alternative heating sources have been shown to be beneficial for inner-city children with asthma.[8]

Elimination of indoor allergens and improving home conditions have also shown to improve asthma outcome in inner-city population.[14,90] In the ICAS, comprehensive environmental control by eliminating home allergens and ETS exposure demonstrated enduring decrease in asthma symptoms and unscheduled asthma visits up to 12 months after cessation of the active intervention.[14] This result emphasizes that environmental allergens and ETS are important factors of asthma control in inner-city children. Improving home conditions, such as home winterization, can decrease mold and moisture exposure and also lead to improved asthma control.[90]

School-Based Interventions

The importance of school-based asthma programs in inner-city asthma care cannot be underestimated, especially in places where transportation to clinics is limited. School-based Asthma Management Program (SAMPRO)[91] contributes asthma education for children, families, clinicians, and school nurses. This program allows multidirectional communications between children and their families, health care providers, and schools. The aim of the program is to encourage better asthma care for children within the school environment by supplying asthma action plans and asthma emergency plans to the school staff.

Other school-based intervention such as Asthma Self-Management for Adolescents (ASMA) provides asthma education for Hispanic and African American adolescents with moderate persistent asthma during the school day. ASMA-enrolled students reported fewer daytime and nighttime asthma symptoms and reduced asthma morbidity and UC usage.[92]

Technology-Based Interventions

Technology-based interventions (text messaging, computer/Web-based, and interactive voice response) are being used to support inner-city asthma care. Of these, only computer/Web-based programs have been successful in reducing asthma symptoms in inner-city children with asthma. Puff City is a Web-based asthma management program designed to improve asthma control in inner-city adolescent with asthma in Detroit, Michigan. Teenagers enrolled in the program experienced fewer ED visits from asthma.[93]

SUMMARY

Inner-city asthma is a complex medical problem with multiple risk factors contributing to high morbidity and mortality. Of these risk factors, allergen sensitization/exposure, ETS exposure, and pollutants are considered to have the most impact on inner-city children with asthma. Other distinctive risk factors of inner-city asthmatics involve poverty and socioeconomic hardship. These factors include poor housing quality, inability to access proper health care, and poor adherence to medications and complicate care for inner-city children with asthma.

Several interventions have shown positive outcome for inner-city children with asthma; however, many of these interventions may not be easily available in real practice settings. These interventions include comprehensive control of home allergens and ETS exposure, the use of anti-IgE monoclonal antibody to prevent seasonal asthma exacerbations, school-based asthma programs, and technology-based initiatives. Future sustainable and expandable interventions in real clinical practice settings are the next targets for inner-city physicians treating children with asthma.

REFERENCES

1. Busse WW, Mitchell H. Addressing issues of asthma in inner-city children. J Allergy Clin Immunol 2007;119(1):43–9.
2. Moorman JE, Akinbami LJ, Bailey CM, et al. National surveillance of asthma: United States, 2001-2010. Vital Health Stat 3 2012;(35):1–58.
3. Keet CA, McCormack MC, Pollack CE, et al. Neighborhood poverty, urban residence, race/ethnicity, and asthma: rethinking the inner-city asthma epidemic. J Allergy Clin Immunol 2015;135(3):655–62.
4. Zahran HS, Bailey CM, Damon SA, et al. Vital signs: asthma in children - United States, 2001-2016. MMWR Morb Mortal Wkly Rep 2018;67(5):149–55.
5. Centers for Disease Control and Prevention. National asthma mortality 2016. Most recent asthma data 2018. Available at: https://www.cdc.gov/asthma/most_recent_data.htm. Accessed May 16, 2018.
6. Busse WW. The National Institutes of Allergy and Infectious Diseases networks on asthma in inner-city children: an approach to improved care. J Allergy Clin Immunol 2010;125(3):529–37 [quiz: 538–9].
7. Liu AH, Babineau DC, Krouse RZ, et al. Pathways through which asthma risk factors contribute to asthma severity in inner-city children. J Allergy Clin Immunol 2016;138(4):1042–50.
8. Poowuttikul P, Saini S, Seth D. Inner-city asthma in children. Clin Rev Allergy Immunol 2019;56(2):248–68.
9. Rosenstreich DL, Eggleston P, Kattan M, et al. The role of cockroach allergy and exposure to cockroach allergen in causing morbidity among inner-city children with asthma. N Engl J Med 1997;336(19):1356–63.
10. Kanchongkittiphon W, Gaffin JM, Phipatanakul W. The indoor environment and inner-city childhood asthma. Asian Pac J Allergy Immunol 2014;32(2):103–10.
11. Sheehan WJ, Rangsithienchai PA, Wood RA, et al. Pest and allergen exposure and abatement in inner-city asthma: a work group report of the American Academy of Allergy, Asthma & Immunology Indoor Allergy/Air Pollution Committee. J Allergy Clin Immunol 2010;125(3):575–81.
12. Cohn RD, Arbes SJ, Jaramillo R, et al. National prevalence and exposure risk for cockroach allergen in U.S. households. Environ Health Perspect 2006;114(4):522–6.
13. Evans R, Gergen PJ, Mitchell H, et al. A randomized clinical trial to reduce asthma morbidity among inner-city children: results of the National Cooperative Inner-City Asthma Study. J Pediatr 1999;135(3):332–8.
14. Morgan WJ, Crain EF, Gruchalla RS, et al. Results of a home-based environmental intervention among urban children with asthma. N Engl J Med 2004;351(11):1068–80.

15. Targonski PV, Persky VW, Ramekrishnan V. Effect of environmental molds on risk of death from asthma during the pollen season. J Allergy Clin Immunol 1995; 95(5 Pt 1):955–61.

16. Wang J, Visness CM, Calatroni A, et al. Effect of environmental allergen sensitization on asthma morbidity in inner-city asthmatic children. Clin Exp Allergy 2009; 39(9):1381–9.

17. O'connor GT, Walter M, Mitchell H, et al. Airborne fungi in the homes of children with asthma in low-income urban communities: the Inner-City Asthma Study. J Allergy Clin Immunol 2004;114(3):599–606.

18. Baxi SN, Muilenberg ML, Rogers CA, et al. Exposures to molds in school classrooms of children with asthma. Pediatr Allergy Immunol 2013;24(7):697–703.

19. Kercsmar CM, Dearborn DG, Schluchter M, et al. Reduction in asthma morbidity in children as a result of home remediation aimed at moisture sources. Environ Health Perspect 2006;114(10):1574–80.

20. Call RS, Smith TF, Morris E, et al. Risk factors for asthma in inner city children. J Pediatr 1992;121(6):862–6.

21. Arlian LG, Bernstein D, Bernstein IL, et al. Prevalence of dust mites in the homes of people with asthma living in eight different geographic areas of the United States. J Allergy Clin Immunol 1992;90(3 Pt 1):292–300.

22. Rabito FA, Iqbal S, Holt E, et al. Prevalence of indoor allergen exposures among New Orleans children with asthma. J Urban Health 2007;84(6):782–92.

23. Chan-Yeung M, Manfreda J, Dimich-Ward H, et al. Mite and cat allergen levels in homes and severity of asthma. Am J Respir Crit Care Med 1995;152(6 Pt 1): 1805–11.

24. Turyk M, Curtis L, Scheff P, et al. Environmental allergens and asthma morbidity in low-income children. J Asthma 2006;43(6):453–7.

25. Matsui EC. Management of rodent exposure and allergy in the pediatric population. Curr Allergy Asthma Rep 2013;13(6):681–6.

26. Phipatanakul W, Eggleston PA, Wright EC, et al. Mouse allergen. I. The prevalence of mouse allergen in inner-city homes. the National Cooperative Inner-City Asthma Study. J Allergy Clin Immunol 2000;106(6):1070–4.

27. Phipatanakul W, Celedón JC, Sredl DL, et al. Mouse exposure and wheeze in the first year of life. Ann Allergy Asthma Immunol 2005;94(5):593–9.

28. Phipatanakul W, Celedón JC, Hoffman EB, et al. Mouse allergen exposure, wheeze and atopy in the first seven years of life. Allergy 2008;63(11):1512–8.

29. Donohue KM, Al-alem U, Perzanowski MS, et al. Anti-cockroach and anti-mouse IgE are associated with early wheeze and atopy in an inner-city birth cohort. J Allergy Clin Immunol 2008;122(5):914–20.

30. Ahluwalia SK, Peng RD, Breysse PN, et al. Mouse allergen is the major allergen of public health relevance in Baltimore City. J Allergy Clin Immunol 2013;132(4): 830–5.e1-2.

31. Matsui EC, Eggleston PA, Buckley TJ, et al. Household mouse allergen exposure and asthma morbidity in inner-city preschool children. Ann Allergy Asthma Immunol 2006;97(4):514–20.

32. Sheehan WJ, Permaul P, Petty CR, et al. Association between allergen exposure in inner-city schools and asthma morbidity among students. JAMA Pediatr 2017; 171(1):31–8.

33. Sheehan WJ, Rangsithienchai PA, Muilenberg ML, et al. Mouse allergens in urban elementary schools and homes of children with asthma. Ann Allergy Asthma Immunol 2009;102(2):125–30.

34. Pongracic JA, Visness CM, Gruchalla RS, et al. Effect of mouse allergen and rodent environmental intervention on asthma in inner-city children. Ann Allergy Asthma Immunol 2008;101(1):35–41.

35. Arbes SJ, Cohn RD, Yin M, et al. Dog allergen (Can f 1) and cat allergen (Fel d 1) in US homes: results from the National Survey of Lead and Allergens in Housing. J Allergy Clin Immunol 2004;114(1):111–7.

36. Gaffin JM, Spergel JM, Boguniewicz M, et al. Effect of cat and daycare exposures on the risk of asthma in children with atopic dermatitis. Allergy Asthma Proc 2012; 33(3):282–8.

37. Kerkhof M, Wijga AH, Brunekreef B, et al. Effects of pets on asthma development up to 8 years of age: the PIAMA study. Allergy 2009;64(8):1202–8.

38. Wegienka G, Johnson CC, Havstad S, et al. Indoor pet exposure and the outcomes of total IgE and sensitization at age 18 years. J Allergy Clin Immunol 2010;126(2):274–9, 279.e271-275.

39. Wegienka G, Johnson CC, Havstad S, et al. Lifetime dog and cat exposure and dog- and cat-specific sensitization at age 18 years. Clin Exp Allergy 2011;41(7): 979–86.

40. McHugh BM, MacGinnitie AJ. Indoor allergen sensitization and the risk of asthma and eczema in children in Pittsburgh. Allergy Asthma Proc 2011;32(5):372–6.

41. Gent JF, Belanger K, Triche EW, et al. Association of pediatric asthma severity with exposure to common household dust allergens. Environ Res 2009;109(6): 768–74.

42. Gent JF, Kezik JM, Hill ME, et al. Household mold and dust allergens: exposure, sensitization and childhood asthma morbidity. Environ Res 2012;118:86–93.

43. Gergen PJ, Mitchell HE, Calatroni A, et al. Sensitization and exposure to pets: the effect on asthma morbidity in the US population. J Allergy Clin Immunol Pract 2018;6(1):101–7.e2.

44. Murray CS, Poletti G, Kebadze T, et al. Study of modifiable risk factors for asthma exacerbations: virus infection and allergen exposure increase the risk of asthma hospital admissions in children. Thorax 2006;61(5):376–82.

45. DiMango E, Serebrisky D, Narula S, et al. Individualized household allergen intervention lowers allergen level but not asthma medication use: a randomized controlled trial. J Allergy Clin Immunol Pract 2016;4(4):671–9.e4.

46. Iwane MK, Prill MM, Lu X, et al. Human rhinovirus species associated with hospitalizations for acute respiratory illness in young US children. J Infect Dis 2011; 204(11):1702–10.

47. Jackson DJ, Gern JE, Lemanske RF. Lessons learned from birth cohort studies conducted in diverse environments. J Allergy Clin Immunol 2017;139(2):379–86.

48. Thorne PS, Kulhánková K, Yin M, et al. Endotoxin exposure is a risk factor for asthma: the national survey of endotoxin in United States housing. Am J Respir Crit Care Med 2005;172(11):1371–7.

49. Sheehan WJ, Hoffman EB, Fu C, et al. Endotoxin exposure in inner-city schools and homes of children with asthma. Ann Allergy Asthma Immunol 2012;108(6): 418–22.

50. Lai PS, Sheehan WJ, Gaffin JM, et al. School endotoxin exposure and asthma morbidity in inner-city children. Chest 2015;148(5):1251–8.

51. Gergen PJ, Teach SJ, Togias A, et al. reducing exacerbations in the inner city: lessons from the inner-city asthma consortium (ICAC). J Allergy Clin Immunol Pract 2016;4(1):22–6.

52. Busse WW, Morgan WJ, Gergen PJ, et al. Randomized trial of omalizumab (anti-IgE) for asthma in inner-city children. N Engl J Med 2011;364(11):1005–15.

53. Teach SJ, Gill MA, Togias A, et al. Preseasonal treatment with either omalizumab or an inhaled corticosteroid boost to prevent fall asthma exacerbations. J Allergy Clin Immunol 2015;136(6):1476–85.

54. Guarnieri M, Balmes JR. Outdoor air pollution and asthma. Lancet 2014; 383(9928):1581–92.

55. Mortimer KM, Neas LM, Dockery DW, et al. The effect of air pollution on inner-city children with asthma. Eur Respir J 2002;19(4):699–705.

56. United States Environmental Protection Agency. Criteria air pollutants 2018. Available at: https://www.epa.gov/criteria-air-pollutants. Accessed June 25, 2018.

57. Matsui EC, Hansel NN, McCormack MC, et al. Asthma in the inner city and the indoor environment. Immunol Allergy Clin North Am 2008;28(3):665–86, x.

58. Permaul P, Phipatanakul W. School environmental intervention programs. J Allergy Clin Immunol Pract 2018;6(1):22–9.

59. Burke H, Leonardi-Bee J, Hashim A, et al. Prenatal and passive smoke exposure and incidence of asthma and wheeze: systematic review and meta-analysis. Pediatrics 2012;129(4):735–44.

60. O'Connor GT, Lynch SV, Bloomberg GR, et al. Early-life home environment and risk of asthma among inner-city children. J Allergy Clin Immunol 2018;141(4): 1468–75.

61. Wang Z, May SM, Charoenlap S, et al. Effects of secondhand smoke exposure on asthma morbidity and health care utilization in children: a systematic review and meta-analysis. Ann Allergy Asthma Immunol 2015;115(5):396–401.e2.

62. Jacob P 3rd, Benowitz NL, Destaillats H, et al. Thirdhand smoke: new evidence, challenges, and future directions. Chem Res Toxicol 2017;30(1):270–94.

63. Godwin C, Batterman S. Indoor air quality in Michigan schools. Indoor Air 2007; 17(2):109–21.

64. Hansel NN, Breysse PN, McCormack MC, et al. A longitudinal study of indoor nitrogen dioxide levels and respiratory symptoms in inner-city children with asthma. Environ Health Perspect 2008;116(10):1428–32.

65. Bauman LJ, Wright E, Leickly FE, et al. Relationship of adherence to pediatric asthma morbidity among inner-city children. Pediatrics 2002;110(1 Pt 1):e6.

66. Szefler SJ, Mitchell H, Sorkness CA, et al. Management of asthma based on exhaled nitric oxide in addition to guideline-based treatment for inner-city adolescents and young adults: a randomised controlled trial. Lancet 2008;372(9643): 1065–72.

67. Poowuttikul P, Hart B, Thomas R, et al. Poor adherence with medication refill and medical supplies maintenance as risk factors for inpatient asthma admission in children. Glob Pediatr Health 2017;4. 2333794X17710588.

68. Michalopoulou G, Briller S, Myers-Schim S, et al. Teaching about better family-clinician partnerships in high-risk pediatric asthma care. J Patient Exp 2016; 3(3):96–9.

69. Dutmer CM, Kim H, Searing DA, et al. Asthma in inner city children: recent insights: United States. Curr Opin Allergy Clin Immunol 2018;18(2):139–47.

70. Ramratnam SK, Visness CM, Jaffee KF, et al. Relationships among maternal stress and depression, type 2 responses, and recurrent wheezing at age 3 years in low-income urban families. Am J Respir Crit Care Med 2017;195(5):674–81.

71. Wing R, Gjelsvik A, Nocera M, et al. Association between adverse childhood experiences in the home and pediatric asthma. Ann Allergy Asthma Immunol 2015; 114(5):379–84.

72. Litonjua AA, Weiss ST. Is vitamin D deficiency to blame for the asthma epidemic? J Allergy Clin Immunol 2007;120(5):1031–5.

73. Freishtat RJ, Iqbal SF, Pillai DK, et al. High prevalence of vitamin D deficiency among inner-city African American youth with asthma in Washington, DC. J Pediatr 2010;156(6):948–52.

74. Vahdaninia M, Mackenzie H, Helps S, et al. Prenatal intake of vitamins and allergic outcomes in the offspring: a systematic review and meta-analysis. J Allergy Clin Immunol Pract 2017;5(3):771–8.e5.

75. Gergen PJ, Togias A. Inner city asthma. Immunol Allergy Clin North Am 2015; 35(1):101–14.

76. Belamarich PF, Luder E, Kattan M, et al. Do obese inner-city children with asthma have more symptoms than nonobese children with asthma? Pediatrics 2000; 106(6):1436–41.

77. Kattan M, Kumar R, Bloomberg GR, et al. Asthma control, adiposity, and adipokines among inner-city adolescents. J Allergy Clin Immunol 2010;125(3):584–92.

78. Jensen ME, Gibson PG, Collins CE, et al. Diet-induced weight loss in obese children with asthma: a randomized controlled trial. Clin Exp Allergy 2013;43(7): 775–84.

79. Gern JE. The urban environment and childhood asthma study. J Allergy Clin Immunol 2010;125(3):545–9.

80. Bousquet J, Gern JE, Martinez FD, et al. Birth cohorts in asthma and allergic diseases: report of a NIAID/NHLBI/MeDALL joint workshop. J Allergy Clin Immunol 2014;133(6):1535–46.

81. Rinas U, Horneff G, Wahn V. Interferon-gamma production by cord-blood mononuclear cells is reduced in newborns with a family history of atopic disease and is independent from cord blood IgE-levels. Pediatr Allergy Immunol 1993;4(2):60–4.

82. Sullivan Dillie KT, Tisler CJ, Dasilva DF, et al. The influence of processing factors and non-atopy-related maternal and neonate characteristics on yield and cytokine responses of cord blood mononuclear cells. Clin Exp Allergy 2008;38(2): 298–304.

83. Pfefferle PI, Büchele G, Blümer N, et al. Cord blood cytokines are modulated by maternal farming activities and consumption of farm dairy products during pregnancy: the PASTURE Study. J Allergy Clin Immunol 2010;125(1):108–15.e1-3.

84. Eder W, Ege MJ, von Mutius E. The asthma epidemic. N Engl J Med 2006; 355(21):2226–35.

85. Yang IV, Pedersen BS, Liu AH, et al. The nasal methylome and childhood atopic asthma. J Allergy Clin Immunol 2017;139(5):1478–88.

86. Esquivel A, Busse WW, Calatroni A, et al. Effects of omalizumab on rhinovirus infections, illnesses, and exacerbations of asthma. Am J Respir Crit Care Med 2017;196(8):985–92.

87. Gill MA, Liu AH, Calatroni A, et al. Enhanced plasmacytoid dendritic cell antiviral responses after omalizumab. J Allergy Clin Immunol 2018;141(5):1735–43.e9.

88. Durham SR, Till SJ. Immunologic changes associated with allergen immunotherapy. J Allergy Clin Immunol 1998;102(2):157–64.

89. Wood RA, Togias A, Wildfire J, et al. Development of cockroach immunotherapy by the inner-city asthma consortium. J Allergy Clin Immunol 2014;133(3): 846–52.e6.

90. Breysse J, Dixon S, Gregory J, et al. Effect of weatherization combined with community health worker in-home education on asthma control. Am J Public Health 2014;104(1):e57–64.

91. Lemanske RF, Kakumanu S, Shanovich K, et al. Creation and implementation of SAMPRO™: a school-based asthma management program. J Allergy Clin Immunol 2016;138(3):711–23.

92. Bruzzese JM, Sheares BJ, Vincent EJ, et al. Effects of a school-based intervention for urban adolescents with asthma. A controlled trial. Am J Respir Crit Care Med 2011;183(8):998–1006.

93. Joseph CLM, Mahajan P, Stokes-Buzzelli S, et al. Pilot study of a randomized trial to evaluate a Web-based intervention targeting adolescents presenting to the emergency department with acute asthma. Pilot Feasibility Stud 2018;4:5.

Allergic Rhinitis in Children and Adolescents

Charles Frank Schuler IV, MD*, Jenny Maribel Montejo, MD

KEYWORDS

- Allergic rhinitis • Immunotherapy • Allergic rhinoconjunctivitis • Allergy
- Prevention of allergic sensitization

KEY POINTS

- Allergic rhinitis is a common disorder that frequently occurs in children and adolescents and carries a high burden of disease.
- Allergic rhinitis can be classified according to severity and timing of symptoms.
- There are several seasonal and perennial triggers of allergic rhinitis, including airborne pollens, molds, dust mites, and animals.
- Avoidance, medications, and immunotherapy may play a role in treating allergic rhinitis.
- Immunotherapy in allergic rhinitis can prevent development of further allergic sensitizations and asthma.

INTRODUCTION

Definition

Allergic rhinitis (AR) is defined as a chronic, waxing/waning, immunoglobulin E (IgE) -based inflammation in the nasopharynx that occurs in response to typically innocuous environmental proteins.[1] Typical symptoms include nasal congestion, rhinorrhea (anterior and/or posterior), sneezing, and itching.[1] When ocular symptoms are included, the disease may be called allergic rhinoconjunctivitis (ARC). This article focuses primarily on AR but will include comments on ARC where relevant.

Epidemiology

AR is a common disease. Typical incidence reports are between 10% and 30% of children and adults in the United States and other developed nations.[2,3] Surveys that specifically use physician-diagnosed AR report rates of approximately 13% in children.[4] Most individuals develop AR symptoms before 20 years of age, with nearly half of such patients becoming symptomatic by age 6 years[5] (**Fig. 1**).

Disclosure Statement: The authors have nothing to disclose.
Division of Allergy and Clinical Immunology, University of Michigan, Domino's Farms, 24 Frank Lloyd Wright Drive, PO Box 442, Suite H-2100, Ann Arbor, MI 48105, USA
* Corresponding author.
E-mail address: schulerc@med.umich.edu

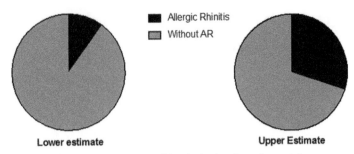

Fig. 1. AR prevalence estimate range worldwide in developed countries.

Indeed, in school-aged children aged 6 to 7, prevalence globally has been reported greater than 8.5%.[6] In adolescents aged 13 to 14, prevalence globally has been reported greater than 14%.[6] Thus, although many patients may develop symptoms at older ages, this is indeed a disease of childhood that can present early in development.

Burden of disease

Furthermore, AR may carry a heavy burden of disease. Symptoms include fatigue, attention, learning, and memory deficits, and even depression.[4,7–9] Nasal obstruction resulting from AR has been shown to contribute to sleep-disordered breathing and can be particularly disruptive of continuous positive airway pressure adherence in patients with obstructive sleep apnea.[10,11] Furthermore, patients with AR may experience a 2-fold increase in medication costs and nearly a 2-fold increase in physician visits.[12] Overall, adolescents with AR and ARC have worse quality of life, which is associated with more nasal symptoms and nasal obstruction as well as reductions in daily functioning and sleep.[13] In addition, there is some evidence that allergic diseases may be more common in patients with attention-deficit/hyperactivity disorder (ADHD), including AR.[14] Treatment of AR is relevant to treatment of ADHD, because treatment of AR reduces ADHD symptom scores.[15]

In addition, AR is consistently associated with asthma. In one population, 38% of patients with AR had asthma, and about 78% of patients with asthma had AR.[16] The additional disease burden of asthma can contribute significantly to patients' difficulty with AR. The authors discuss further how this process might be interrupted using immunotherapy (IT) in later discussion.

Numerous risk factors have been found to predispose to AR. These risk factors include a family history of allergic diseases, male sex, birth during the pollen season, firstborn status, early-life antibiotic use, maternal smoking, indoor allergen exposure, elevated serum IgE levels (>100 IU/mL) before age 6, and any presence of allergen-specific IgE.[17,18]

Diagnostic Considerations

A typical history of AR includes symptoms of sneezing, rhinorrhea, nasal obstruction, and nasal itching. Other common symptoms include cough, postnasal drip, irritability, and fatigue. Some patients also describe palate and inner ear itching. ARC may include ocular symptoms, such as ocular itching, tearing, and burning. Younger children may exhibit different symptoms, such as snorting or sniffing, throat clearing, and cough. To scratch an itchy palate, children may make a clicking sound as they move the tongue against the palate to relieve this pruritic sensation.[19–21] Symptoms may be present year-round or seasonally, depending on the timing of allergen exposures.

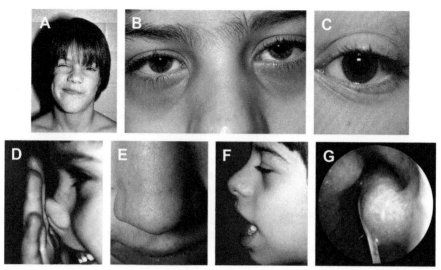

Fig. 2. The pathophysiology of AR results in typical examination findings illustrated here. See text for full descriptions. (*A*) Facial grimacing or twitching. This is related to nasal itching. (*B*) Allergic shiners. (*C*) Dennie-Morgan lines. (*D*) The allergic salute. (*E*) Nasal creasing related to the allergic salute. (*F*) Allergic facies. (*G*) Typical nasal mucosa. (*From* Chong H, Green T, Larkin A. Allergy and Immunology. In: Zitelli, B., McIntire, S. and Nowalk, A. (2018). Zitelli and Davis' Atlas of Pediatric Physical Diagnosis. Philadelphia: Elsevier, pp.108-109; with permission.)

Patients may be able to identify triggers, such as pet exposure, or a specific time of year when symptoms worsen, and it can be helpful to elicit these history points to guide avoidance measures (discussed later).

a. Typical examination findings include the following (**Fig. 2**)[19]:
   i. Allergic shiners: These occur because of infraorbital edema from venodilation related to blood vessel changes in the context of allergic inflammation.
   ii. Dennie-Morgan lines: These consist of increased folds or lines below the lower eyelid and are more common in patients with AR. The pathophysiology is not precisely understood. These lines do not always denote AR and can be more common in some ethnic groups without an increase in AR.
   iii. Allergic salute: This is a behavior related to nasal itching and rhinorrhea consisting of repeated rubbing of the nose. This repeated pushing the tip of the nose up with the hand leads to a transverse nasal crease.
   iv. Allergic facies: Typical allergic facies consist of a high arched palate, mouth breathing, and dental malocclusion. This is generally seen in children with early-onset AR.
   v. Nasal mucosa: With anterior rhinoscopy, the nasal mucosa may appear pale and blue colored with turbinate edema. This may be accompanied by visible clear rhinorrhea (anterior or posterior in oropharynx).
   vi. Cobblestoning: The posterior oropharynx may develop hyperplastic lymphoid tissue leading to a "cobblestone" appearance of the mucosa.
   vii. The tympanic membranes may also be abnormal, either with retraction or with serous fluid accumulation. This is related to nasal mucosal swelling and eustachian tube dysfunction.[22]
b. Specific IgE testing

Once the diagnosis of AR is suggested by the history and examination, determining specific IgE positivity may be helpful to confirm the diagnosis. Determination of specific IgE is indicated when it is necessary to establish an allergic cause for the patient's symptoms, to confirm or exclude specific allergic causes for a patient's symptoms, or to determine specific allergen sensitivity to guide avoidance measures or IT.[19] Skin testing to specific antigens can be done safely in the allergy office and provides results within 20 minutes with good sensitivity and specificity. Specific blood IgE testing has similar sensitivity to skin testing when considering patients with nasal allergic reactions upon allergen challenge testing.[19] The authors generally prefer skin testing in children because of the rapid results (20 minutes), lack of need for blood and laboratory-associated processing time, and ability to perform counseling in the same visit as testing based on real-time results. Anecdotally, patients and families appreciate this real-time diagnostic approach.

Allergic Rhinitis Classification

Once the diagnosis of AR is made, the disease can be classified according to whether it is intermittent or persistent as well as based on severity.[23] Intermittent AR is defined as having symptoms present for less than 4 weeks and for less than 4 days per week. Persistent AR occurs when symptoms are present for greater than 4 weeks and greater than 4 days per week.

Severity of disease can be classified according to the following:

a. Mild: Does not meet definition of moderate/severe
b. Moderate/severe: Meets one or more of the following criteria:
    i. Sleep disturbance
    ii. Impairment of school/work performance
    iii. Impairment of daily activities, leisure, or sports involvement
    iv. Troublesome symptoms

In practice, AR is often divided into seasonal and perennial subtypes as well, because this tends to relate to the allergic sensitizations specific to the patient.[1,19] Persistent or perennial symptoms tend to be more common than isolated seasonal symptoms, although a mixed picture, with persistent symptoms coupled with seasonal exacerbations, is quite common.[24] Many patients will lose awareness of the disability associated with AR if chronic symptoms are present. Children are particularly vulnerable to ignoring severe symptoms when present for prolonged periods. Lack of symptom awareness can have a profoundly detrimental effect on school/examination performance and contributes to the burden of disease described previously.[25–27]

Triggers

Triggers of AR are divided according to their temporal pattern during the year, as either perennial or seasonal triggers. Perennial triggers include items present in the home year round, such as mold, dust mites, or animals (particularly cats and dogs). Some patients also have perennial symptoms from an occupational exposure.[28] Thus, a thorough environmental history can be helpful in identifying potential control or avoidance measures that might improve perennial symptom control. Typical history might include visible mold presence in the home, presence of animals, bedding and other dust mite exposures, occupation, and hobbies. This information can be useful in guiding avoidance measures, detailed in later discussion.

Seasonal triggers include various pollens and molds. The typical pollens involved are tree, grass, and weed species that pollinate via wind-based pollen distribution.

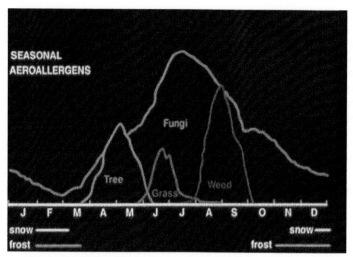

Fig. 3. Representative seasonal aeroallergen counts for Ann Arbor, MI. (*Courtesy of* WR. Solomon, MD, Ann Arbor, MI.)

A representative pollen count is displayed (**Fig. 3**) based on data historically collected in the authors' local area by Dr Bill Solomon. Correlating symptoms with pollen counts can give insight into the cause of a patient's seasonal symptoms. Insect-pollinated plants are not as commonly implicated in AR disease pathogenesis because of the lack of diffuse airborne pollen dispersal in these plants' life cycles. Some colloquial names for seasonal allergies identify times of the year with an event. However, physicians should be aware that the name may not identify the actual culprit pollinating species. For example, one colloquial name for AR is rose fever. This name correctly identifies that symptoms occur in early summer when rose blooming occurs. However, the rhinitis symptoms associated with the name is actually from pollinating grasses. Another classic example is the term hay fever. This term notes symptoms that occur during the fall hay harvest. However, the actual culprit allergens are more likely mold growing on the hay or weed pollens disseminated during the fall that contribute to rhinitis.

Therapy

Therapy for AR can be conceptualized as a 3-pronged approach. This approach includes avoidance, medications, and IT. Each aspect of therapy is discussed in detail. Special focus is given to the prevention of the development of other allergic sensitizations and asthma with IT in this section.

a. Avoidance: Success in avoidance of a culprit allergen is best measured by measuring the reduction in symptoms and medication use rather than a change in allergen concentration.[29] Each type of specific allergen is dealt with in later discussion.
  i. Dust mite: Dust mite feces are a major allergenic source in house dust, and the principal food of dust mites is human skin.[30,31] Major reservoirs of dust mite include mattresses, bedding, and upholstery. In general, a combination of multiple measures has been found to be most effective in mitigating symptoms from dust mite exposure. Typically, this includes dust mite covers for bedding, humidity control (between 35% and 50%) of the ambient air in the home, HEPA

vacuuming of carpet, and acaricides.[32] Using only a single measure to attempt to mitigate dust mite exposure does not seem to be effective. For example, using mite-proof bedding alone may not be sufficient for dust mite control.[32] In practice, patients and families may have difficulty implementing a full dust mite regimen, and physicians should be aware that partial implementation may not lead to dramatic symptom improvement.

ii. Animals: Total animal avoidance is thought to be the most effective way to improve symptoms.[19] Anecdotally, it is the opinion of the authors that it can be very hard for patients and families to remove animals from the home; if total home avoidance is to be accomplished, it must often be done prospectively rather than after an animal has joined a family. If the animal must remain in the house, the combination of a HEPA filter, mattress/pillow covers, and animal removal from the bedroom has been shown to reduce airborne antigen but not clinical symptoms in asthma; the effect on AR is less clear.[33] This underlines the difficulty of mitigating the continued presence of a pet. Furthermore, in counseling patients about possible new pets, hypoallergenic pets are not thought to actually exist, as even animals engineered to not produce a major allergen will still produce other allergens from the species, which can still elicit symptoms.[34] There is observational evidence that living with an animal during the first year of life may reduce the risk of developing sensitization to cat or dog in the future.[35,36] This suggests that avoiding animal purchases before a member of the household develops AR will not prevent allergy, but actually quite the opposite.

iii. Pollen: Avoidance of pollens during the season is very difficult because of their airborne ubiquity. Suggested measures include keeping windows closed, staying indoors on high-pollen days if highly allergic, avoiding drying clothing outside, and showering before bed to reduce carrying pollens through the night.[19]

iv. Mold: Avoidance measures for mold primarily focus on reducing indoor exposure. Suggested measures include reducing moisture sources, removing contaminated items from the home, applying diluted bleach to molds growing in the home on nonporous surfaces, wearing face masks for exposure to soil, leaves, compost, increasing air circulation, and cleaning air conditioning units regularly.[19]

b. Medications: Numerous medications have been developed to treat AR. These medications generally treat only symptoms and do not address the underlying allergic inflammation. Nevertheless, medical management of AR can be quite effective at mitigating the negative effects of the disease.

i. Nasal irrigation: Nasal saline irrigation, typically performed once daily, has shown benefit in AR. The practice led to improved symptoms and nasal peak flows in pediatric patients in one randomized placebo-controlled study.[37] Nasal irrigation may also serve as an adjunctive therapy that could decrease the need for nasal steroid dosing, because it improved symptoms and mucociliary clearance in children also on nasal steroids in a separate study.[38]

ii. Antihistamines: Oral antihistamines are used in AR to target the H1 receptor. This can effectively reduce symptoms of rhinorrhea, sneezing, and nasal itching.[39] First-generation H1 antihistamines, such as diphenhydramine, tend to cross the blood-brain barrier and induce sedation partly via an anticholinergic action.[40] Cumulative use over the lifetime has previously been associated with risk of dementia based on this anticholinergic property set.[41] Second-generation oral antihistamines, such as fexofenadine or cetirizine, appear to have similar effectiveness as first-generation H1 antihistamines without evidence of the same risk profile because of the lack of brain penetration.[42] Fexofenadine and cetirizine are approved for children older than 6 months old and are an important tool in the AR armamentarium in children.

iii. Intranasal steroids: Intranasal steroids (NS) demonstrate excellent evidence toward anti-inflammatory properties that reduce rhinorrhea, itching, sneezing, and nasal obstruction or congestion.[43,44] Some limited evidence exists to suggest that NS reduce ocular symptoms of ARC as well, such as tearing, redness, itching, and swelling.[45] Overall, NS are thought to be the most effective single pharmaceutical in AR.[46] Mometasone, fluticasone, and triamcinolone nasal sprays are approved for children older than 2 years old. Adherence in small children especially can be troublesome. The authors find that choosing NS varieties with minimal volume and scent seems to help children tolerate these drugs.

iv. Intranasal antihistamines: Intranasal antihistamines also work on the H1 receptor and show similar effects to oral antihistamines; in fact, they may significantly reduce symptoms.[46] They are thought to achieve higher drug levels in nasal tissues and thus have a true anti-inflammatory effect, such as mast cell stabilization, not present with oral antihistamines.[47] Azelastine nasal spray is approved for children older than 5 years old. Adherence is an issue in children, because side effects may include bitter taste and sedation.[48] The bitter taste in particular can make it difficult for small children to tolerate the medication.

v. Leukotriene modifiers: Leukotrienes are inflammatory mediators related to AR pathogenesis. Leukotriene modifiers block the cysteinyl leukotriene receptor. Montelukast is approved in the United States for children 6 months and older and is effective at relieving AR symptoms; it also has a good safety profile.[49] Because montelukast is approved for both asthma and AR in children, it is often a good choice in patients with both diseases.[49] Physicians should be aware of the postmarketing data suggesting that montelukast may be detrimental in mood and be related to suicidality. However, the association is weak and thought to be very rare, and with proper counseling and monitoring, the use of the drug need not be limited.[50,51]

c. Immunotherapy: IT involves giving patients extracts containing allergens to which they produce specific IgE in order to induce immune changes and a desensitized state. Various formulations have been tried, but the most widely used at this time are subcutaneous injections and sublingual applications. Only these two are discussed in this section.

i. Subcutaneous immunotherapy: Subcutaneous immunotherapy (or "SCIT," often pronounced "skit") consists of injecting a patient with diluted extracts of the allergens that are thought to exacerbate the patient's AR. Very dilute extracts are used to start, and these are gradually escalated to higher concentrations, usually on a weekly schedule that requires several months of regular adherence. Once the highest concentration is achieved, this is called "maintenance," and the interval between injects can be lengthened. SCIT directly affects the immune system and changes the response to allergen. The details of this process are listed in **Table 1**. There is some disagreement surrounding whether multiple allergens should be combined or whether only a single relevant allergen should be administered at 1 time; this discussion is beyond the scope of this article.

1. Indications: Current guidelines suggest considering SCIT in AR when patients have evidence of elevated levels of specific IgE to clinically relevant allergens. The applicability to a particular patient should include

Table 1 Immunologic changes associated with subcutaneous immunotherapy and sublingual immunotherapy	
Decrease in humoral and cellular response to allergens	IgE levels to allergen initially increase and then decrease over time
	Allergen-specific IgG1, IgG4, and IgA increase with time (although this does not predict effectiveness of IT)
	Decreased allergen-related eosinophil, basophil, and mast cell infiltration
Decreased end-organ response to allergen	Includes skin, conjunctiva, nasal mucosa, bronchi
	Blunted mucosal priming in response to allergen
	Decrease in bronchial histamine sensitivity
Increasing tolerance of allergen	Increase in regulatory T-cell number and production of interleukin-10 and transforming growth factor-B
	Waning of T-helper 2 (Th2) response and transition to Th1 response to allergen

SLIT is less well studied but thus far shows similar effects.

Data form Cox, L., et al., Allergen immunotherapy: a practice parameter third update. J Allergy Clin Immunol, 2011. **127**(1 Suppl): p. S1-55.

consideration of patient preference, adherence issues, other medication needs, response to avoidance measures, medication adverse effects, and the possibility of preventing allergic asthma in patients with AR (see later discussion).[52]

2. Effectiveness: Multiple double-blind, placebo-controlled, randomized clinical trials show effectiveness for SCIT for AR, and effectiveness of 3 to 5 years of therapy is the best studied.[53] SCIT is effective at ameliorating ocular symptoms as well.[54] Efficacy has been confirmed for pollens, fungi, animal allergens, dust mites, and cockroaches.[52] Improvements typically occur across multiple measurement domains, including symptoms, medication scores, organ challenges, immunologic changes, and quality of life.[52]

ii. Sublingual immunotherapy: Sublingual immunotherapy (or "SLIT") has also been studied in AR. SLIT involves the sublingual application of diluted allergen extracts thought to exacerbate a patient's AR with a similar buildup schedule to SCIT. The mechanism of action is thought to be similar to SCIT (see later discussion). SLIT is less relevant for pediatric patients because of a current lack of available products for children. A Timothy grass pollen extract is approved down to 5 years old. A 5-grass extract is approved down to 10 years old. Dust mite and ragweed extracts are approved only starting at age 18.

1. Indications: SLIT has similar indications to SCIT, although this is less well defined. SLIT can be particularly appropriate for patients who wish to avoid injections. Each product is only approved for single use, not in a combined fashion as SCIT may be used.[55]

2. Effectiveness: Timothy and combined 5-grass tablets have shown improvement in symptom and medication scores in the first year of treatment.[55] Dust mite and ragweed extracts are not approved for patients less than 18 years old. No direct studies between SCIT and SLIT have been done to date.

iii. Avoidance of asthma development with SCIT, avoidance of other sensitizations: SCIT has shown an ability to reduce the risk of asthma development and reduce the risk of developing additional IgE sensitizations. Studies of SLIT have also begun to show this effect. This has implications for interrupting the progression of atopic disease, and IT is one of only a few interventions shown to have this effect on the atopic march. Particularly in children, IT should be considered early in the treatment of AR due to the potentially preventative effects detailed in later discussion.

1. Asthma development: Multiple studies have shown a reduction in asthma development associated with SCIT and SLIT. In 1 study, 3 years of pollen-based SCIT in children with AR reduced the risk of asthma development 2 years after stopping SCIT; this effect persisted at a 10-year follow-up (7 years after stopping SCIT) with an odds ratio of no asthma of 4.6.[56,57] Coseasonal grass SLIT administered for 3 years reduced asthma development versus controls in children aged 5 to 14 years.[58] This has been borne out in a multinational double-blind placebo-controlled setting out to 5 years.[59] Similar effects have been shown using dust mite SLIT, which reduced asthma development and new allergic sensitization in children as well up to 15 years later.[60–63]

2. Further sensitization:
   a. Twelve years after stopping grass SCIT, treated children had a lower rate of new sensitization development versus controls (58% vs 100%).[64]
   b. House dust mite SCIT in children monosensitized to dust mite also reduced the rate of new sensitization to other allergens up to 6 years later.[65–67]
   c. Among all monosensitized AR patients, one retrospective trial of greater than 8000 patients showed a decrease in new sensitization over 7 years in SCIT-treated patients.[68]
   d. Some studies have not shown a difference between SLIT and placebo with respect to new sensitizations with house dust mite SLIT.[69]

SUMMARY

Overall, AR is an allergic disease characterized by nasal symptoms, and when accompanied by ocular symptoms, is called ARC. The disease is common, may start early in life, and is associated with a high burden of disease that can particularly impair the functioning of children in school and other domains of life. Identifying seasonal and perennial triggers can be helpful, and the first step of treating the patient is avoidance. Medications are very helpful for treating symptoms and mitigating the disease burden but do not usually affect the underlying inflammation. IT not only has been shown to improve AR but also may prevent additional allergic sensitizations and asthma development.

REFERENCES

1. Dykewicz MS, Wallace DV, Baroody F, et al. Treatment of seasonal allergic rhinitis: an evidence-based focused 2017 guideline update. Ann Allergy Asthma Immunol 2017;119(6):489–511.e41.

2. Settipane RA. Demographics and epidemiology of allergic and nonallergic rhinitis. Allergy Asthma Proc 2001;22(4):185–9.

3. Singh K, Axelrod S, Bielory L. The epidemiology of ocular and nasal allergy in the United States, 1988-1994. J Allergy Clin Immunol 2010;126(4):778–783 e6.

4. Meltzer EO, Blaiss MS, Naclerio RM, et al. Burden of allergic rhinitis: allergies in America, Latin America, and Asia-Pacific adult surveys. Allergy Asthma Proc 2012;33(Suppl 1):S113–41.

5. Meltzer EO, Blaiss MS, Derebery MJ, et al. Burden of allergic rhinitis: results from the Pediatric Allergies in America survey. J Allergy Clin Immunol 2009; 124(3 Suppl):S43–70.

6. Mallol J, Crane J, von Mutius E, et al. The International Study of Asthma and Allergies in Childhood (ISAAC) phase three: a global synthesis. Allergol Immuno-pathol (Madr) 2013;41(2):73–85.

7. Meltzer EO. Allergic rhinitis: burden of illness, quality of life, comorbidities, and control. Immunol Allergy Clin North Am 2016;36(2):235–48.

8. Muliol J, Maurer M, Bousquet J. Sleep and allergic rhinitis. J Investig Allergol Clin Immunol 2008;18(6):415–9.

9. Colas C, Galera H, Añibarro B, et al. Disease severity impairs sleep quality in allergic rhinitis (The SOMNIAAR study). Clin Exp Allergy 2012;42(7):1080–7.

10. Georgalas C. The role of the nose in snoring and obstructive sleep apnoea: an update. Eur Arch Otorhinolaryngol 2011;268(9):1365–73.

11. Koinis-Mitchell D, Craig T, Esteban CA, et al. Sleep and allergic disease: a sum-mary of the literature and future directions for research. J Allergy Clin Immunol 2012;130(6):1275–81.

12. Nathan RA. The burden of allergic rhinitis. Allergy Asthma Proc 2007;28(1):3–9.

13. Blaiss MS, Hammerby E, Robinson S, et al. The burden of allergic rhinitis and allergic rhinoconjunctivitis on adolescents: a literature review. Ann Allergy Asthma Immunol 2018;121(1):43–52.e3.

14. Miyazaki C, Koyama M, Ota E, et al. Allergic diseases in children with attention deficit hyperactivity disorder: a systematic review and meta-analysis. BMC Psy-chiatry 2017;17(1):120.

15. Yang MT, Chen CC, Lee WT, et al. Attention-deficit/hyperactivity disorder-related symptoms improved with allergic rhinitis treatment in children. Am J Rhinol Allergy 2016;30(3):209–14.

16. Casale TB, Dykewicz MS. Clinical implications of the allergic rhinitis-asthma link. Am J Med Sci 2004;327(3):127–38.

17. Matheson MC, Dharmage SC, Abramson MJ, et al. Early-life risk factors and inci-dence of rhinitis: results from the European Community Respiratory Health Study–an international population-based cohort study. J Allergy Clin Immunol 2011; 128(4):816–823 e5.

18. Saulyte J, Regueira C, Montes-Martínez A, et al. Active or passive exposure to tobacco smoking and allergic rhinitis, allergic dermatitis, and food allergy in adults and children: a systematic review and meta-analysis. PLoS Med 2014; 11(3):e1001611.

19. Wallace DV, Dykewicz MS, Bernstein DI, et al. The diagnosis and management of rhinitis: an updated practice parameter. J Allergy Clin Immunol 2008;122(2 Suppl):S1–84.

20. Ng ML, Warlow RS, Chrishanthan N, et al. Preliminary criteria for the definition of allergic rhinitis: a systematic evaluation of clinical parameters in a disease cohort (I). Clin Exp Allergy 2000;30(9):1314–31.

21. Ng ML, Warlow RS, Chrishanthan N, et al. Preliminary criteria for the definition of allergic rhinitis: a systematic evaluation of clinical parameters in a disease cohort (II). Clin Exp Allergy 2000;30(10):1417–22.

22. Fireman P. Otitis media and eustachian tube dysfunction: connection to allergic rhinitis. J Allergy Clin Immunol 1997;99(2):S787–97.

23. Bousquet J, Van Cauwenberge P, Khaltaev N, Aria Workshop Group, World Health Organization. Allergic rhinitis and its impact on asthma. J Allergy Clin Im-munol 2001;108(5 Suppl):S147–334.

24. Mullarkey MF, Hill JS, Webb DR. Allergic and nonallergic rhinitis: their characterization with attention to the meaning of nasal eosinophilia. J Allergy Clin Immunol 1980;65(2):122–6.

25. Kremer B, den Hartog HM, Jolles J. Relationship between allergic rhinitis, disturbed cognitive functions and psychological well-being. Clin Exp Allergy 2002;32(9):1310–5.

26. Marshall PS, O'Hara C, Steinberg P. Effects of seasonal allergic rhinitis on selected cognitive abilities. Ann Allergy Asthma Immunol 2000;84(4):403–10.

27. Walker S, Khan-Wasti S, Fletcher M, et al. Seasonal allergic rhinitis is associated with a detrimental effect on examination performance in United Kingdom teenagers: case-control study. J Allergy Clin Immunol 2007;120(2):381–7.

28. Siracusa A, Desrosiers M, Marabini A. Epidemiology of occupational rhinitis: prevalence, aetiology and determinants. Clin Exp Allergy 2000;30(11):1519–34.

29. Platts-Mills TA, Thomas WR, Aalberse RC, et al. Dust mite allergens and asthma: report of a second international workshop. J Allergy Clin Immunol 1992;89(5): 1046–60.

30. Park GM, Lee SM, Lee IY, et al. Localization of a major allergen, Der p 2, in the gut and faecal pellets of Dermatophagoides pteronyssinus. Clin Exp Allergy 2000; 30(9):1293–7.

31. Pollart S, Chapman MD, Platts-Mills TA. House dust mite and dust control. Clin Rev Allergy 1988;6(1):23–33.

32. Sheikh A, Hurwitz B, Nurmatov U, et al. House dust mite avoidance measures for perennial allergic rhinitis. Cochrane Database Syst Rev 2010;(7):CD001563.

33. Wood RA, Johnson EF, Van Natta ML, et al. A placebo-controlled trial of a HEPA air cleaner in the treatment of cat allergy. Am J Respir Crit Care Med 1998;158(1): 115–20.

34. Portnoy J, Kennedy K, Sublett J, et al. Environmental assessment and exposure control: a practice parameter–furry animals. Ann Allergy Asthma Immunol 2012; 108(4):223.e1-15.

35. Mandhane PJ, Sears MR, Poulton R, et al. Cats and dogs and the risk of atopy in childhood and adulthood. J Allergy Clin Immunol 2009;124(4):745–750 e4.

36. Wegienka G, Johnson CC, Havstad S, et al. Lifetime dog and cat exposure and dog- and cat-specific sensitization at age 18 years. Clin Exp Allergy 2011;41(7): 979–86.

37. Wang YH, Yang CP, Ku MS, et al. Efficacy of nasal irrigation in the treatment of acute sinusitis in children. Int J Pediatr Otorhinolaryngol 2009;73(12):1696–701.

38. Li H, Sha Q, Zuo K, et al. Nasal saline irrigation facilitates control of allergic rhinitis by topical steroid in children. ORL J Otorhinolaryngol Relat Spec 2009; 71(1):50–5.

39. Simons FE. Advances in H1-antihistamines. N Engl J Med 2004;351(21):2203–17.

40. Church MK, Maurer M, Simons FE, et al. Risk of first-generation H(1)-antihistamines: a GA(2)LEN position paper. Allergy 2010;65(4):459–66.

41. Gray SL, Anderson ML, Dublin S, et al. Cumulative use of strong anticholinergics and incident dementia: a prospective cohort study. JAMA Intern Med 2015; 175(3):401–7.

42. Golightly LK, Greos LS. Second-generation antihistamines: actions and efficacy in the management of allergic disorders. Drugs 2005;65(3):341–84.

43. Rodrigo GJ, Neffen H. Efficacy of fluticasone furoate nasal spray vs. placebo for the treatment of ocular and nasal symptoms of allergic rhinitis: a systematic review. Clin Exp Allergy 2011;41(2):160–70.

44. Penagos M, Compalati E, Tarantini F, et al. Efficacy of mometasone furoate nasal spray in the treatment of allergic rhinitis. Meta-analysis of randomized, double-blind, placebo-controlled, clinical trials. Allergy 2008;63(10):1280–91.

45. Bielory L, Chun Y, Bielory BP, et al. Impact of mometasone furoate nasal spray on individual ocular symptoms of allergic rhinitis: a meta-analysis. Allergy 2011; 66(5):686–93.

46. Benninger M, Farrar JR, Blaiss M, et al. Evaluating approved medications to treat allergic rhinitis in the United States: an evidence-based review of efficacy for nasal symptoms by class. Ann Allergy Asthma Immunol 2010;104(1):13–29.

47. Pipkorn P, Costantini C, Reynolds C, et al. The effects of the nasal antihistamines olopatadine and azelastine in nasal allergen provocation. Ann Allergy Asthma Immunol 2008;101(1):82–9.

48. Lumry W, Prenner B, Corren J, et al. Efficacy and safety of azelastine nasal spray at a dose of 1 spray per nostril twice daily. Ann Allergy Asthma Immunol 2007; 99(3):267–72.

49. Nayak A. A review of montelukast in the treatment of asthma and allergic rhinitis. Expert Opin Pharmacother 2004;5(3):679–86.

50. Philip G, Hustad C, Noonan G, et al. Reports of suicidality in clinical trials of montelukast. J Allergy Clin Immunol 2009;124(4):691–6.e6.

51. Holbrook JT, Harik-Khan R. Montelukast and emotional well-being as a marker for depression: results from 3 randomized, double-masked clinical trials. J Allergy Clin Immunol 2008;122(4):828–9.

52. Cox L, Nelson H, Lockey R, et al. Allergen immunotherapy: a practice parameter third update. J Allergy Clin Immunol 2011;127(1 Suppl):S1–55.

53. Ross RN, Nelson HS, Finegold I. Effectiveness of specific immunotherapy in the treatment of allergic rhinitis: an analysis of randomized, prospective, single- or double-blind, placebo-controlled studies. Clin Ther 2000;22(3):342–50.

54. Lowell FC, Franklin W. A double-blind study of the effectiveness and specificity of injection therapy in ragweed hay fever. N Engl J Med 1965;273(13):675–9.

55. Greenhawt M, Oppenheimer J, Nelson M, et al. Sublingual immunotherapy: a focused allergen immunotherapy practice parameter update. Ann Allergy Asthma Immunol 2017;118(3):276–282 e2.

56. Jacobsen L, Niggemann B, Dreborg S, et al. Specific immunotherapy has long-term preventive effect of seasonal and perennial asthma: 10-year follow-up on the PAT study. Allergy 2007;62(8):943–8.

57. Moller C, Dreborg S, Ferdousi HA, et al. Pollen immunotherapy reduces the development of asthma in children with seasonal rhinoconjunctivitis (the PAT-study). J Allergy Clin Immunol 2002;109(2):251–6.

58. Novembre E, Galli E, Landi F, et al. Coseasonal sublingual immunotherapy reduces the development of asthma in children with allergic rhinoconjunctivitis. J Allergy Clin Immunol 2004;114(4):851–7.

59. Valovirta E, Petersen TH, Piotrowska T, et al. Results from the 5-year SQ grass sublingual immunotherapy tablet asthma prevention (GAP) trial in children with grass pollen allergy. J Allergy Clin Immunol 2018;141(2):529–38.e13.

60. Di Rienzo V, Marcucci F, Puccinelli P, et al. Long-lasting effect of sublingual immunotherapy in children with asthma due to house dust mite: a 10-year prospective study. Clin Exp Allergy 2003;33(2):206–10.

61. Marogna M, Spadolini I, Massolo A, et al. Randomized controlled open study of sublingual immunotherapy for respiratory allergy in real-life: clinical efficacy and more. Allergy 2004;59(11):1205–10.

62. Marogna M, Tomassetti D, Bernasconi A, et al. Preventive effects of sublingual immunotherapy in childhood: an open randomized controlled study. Ann Allergy Asthma Immunol 2008;101(2):206–11.
63. Marogna M, Spadolini I, Massolo A, et al. Long-lasting effects of sublingual immunotherapy according to its duration: a 15-year prospective study. J Allergy Clin Immunol 2010;126(5):969–75.
64. Eng PA, Borer-Reinhold M, Heijnen IA, et al. Twelve-year follow-up after discontinuation of preseasonal grass pollen immunotherapy in childhood. Allergy 2006;61(2):198–201.
65. Des Roches A, Paradis L, Menardo JL, et al. Immunotherapy with a standardized Dermatophagoides pteronyssinus extract. VI. Specific immunotherapy prevents the onset of new sensitizations in children. J Allergy Clin Immunol 1997;99(4):450–3.
66. Pajno GB, Barberio G, De Luca F, et al. Prevention of new sensitizations in asthmatic children monosensitized to house dust mite by specific immunotherapy. A six-year follow-up study. Clin Exp Allergy 2001;31(9):1392–7.
67. Inal A, Altintas DU, Yilmaz M, et al. Prevention of new sensitizations by specific immunotherapy in children with rhinitis and/or asthma monosensitized to house dust mite. J Investig Allergol Clin Immunol 2007;17(2):85–91.
68. Purello-D'Ambrosio F, Gangemi S, Merendino RA, et al. Prevention of new sensitizations in monosensitized subjects submitted to specific immunotherapy or not. A retrospective study. Clin Exp Allergy 2001;31(8):1295–302.
69. Lim JH, Kim JY, Han DH, et al. Sublingual immunotherapy (SLIT) for house dust mites does not prevent new allergen sensitization and bronchial hyperresponsiveness in allergic rhinitis children. PLoS One 2017;12(8):e0182295.

Anaphylaxis in Children and Adolescents

Pavadee Poowuttikul, MD*, Divya Seth, MD

KEYWORDS

- Anaphylaxis • Anaphylactic reaction • Allergic reaction • Anaphylactoid

KEY POINTS

- Anaphylaxis is an acute, potentially life-threatening systemic hypersensitivity reaction that should be recognized promptly.
- Food allergy is the most common cause of anaphylaxis, followed by drugs.
- Signs and symptoms of anaphylaxis include urticaria, angioedema, respiratory distress, nausea, vomiting, diarrhea, and hypotension.
- Up to 10% of patients with anaphylaxis can present without cutaneous findings. This lack of skin/mucosal involvement can lead to misdiagnosis or delayed diagnosis of anaphylaxis.
- Epinephrine is the first drug of choice for treating anaphylaxis. Delayed epinephrine administration is associated with increase in morbidity and mortality.

INTRODUCTION

Anaphylaxis is an acute, potentially life-threatening systemic hypersensitivity reaction. Classically anaphylaxis is an immunoglobulin (Ig) E–mediated reaction; however, IgG or immune complex complement-related immunologic reactions that lead to degranulation of mast cells can also cause anaphylaxis. Food allergy is the most common cause of anaphylaxis, followed by drugs. The most common foods causing anaphylaxis are cow's milk in infants, peanuts in children, and tree nuts and shellfish in young adults. Beta-lactam antibiotics are the most common culprits of drug-induced anaphylaxis.

Patients with anaphylaxis commonly present with symptoms involving skin or mucous membranes, followed by respiratory and gastrointestinal symptoms. By definition, anaphylaxis involves at least 2 body systems. Anaphylaxis is also considered if only hypotension occurs without other clinical findings after exposure to a specific allergen known to the individual.[1–4] Epinephrine is the first drug of choice in treating anaphylaxis. Patients and caregivers should be educated in the use of epinephrine autoinjectors. Delayed epinephrine injection increases the risk of hospitalization and death from anaphylaxis.

Disclosure: The authors have nothing to disclose.
Children's Hospital of Michigan, Wayne State University School of Medicine, 3950 Beaubien, Detroit, MI 48201, USA
* Corresponding author.
E-mail address: ppoowutt@med.wayne.edu

PATHOGENESIS AND CLASSIFICATION

Traditionally anaphylaxis is an IgE-mediated immunologic reaction that leads to the release of mediators from mast cells and basophils; however, IgG (animal models only) and immune complex/complement-mediated immunologic reactions can also cause anaphylaxis.

Nonimmunologic mechanisms such as direct release of mast cell and basophil mediators or complement activation are also known to cause anaphylactic reactions.[2] These non–IgE-mediated or non–immune systemic reactions were previously termed anaphylactoid reactions. However, the World Allergy Organization has categorized anaphylaxis as allergic anaphylaxis, when the reaction is mediated by immune mechanisms (either from IgE, IgG, or immune complex) and nonallergic anaphylaxis, when the reaction is not immunologically mediated, thus eliminating the term anaphylactoid.[5] Both the IgE-mediated and non–IgE-mediated mechanisms release platelet-activating factor, whereas only the IgE-dependent mechanism releases histamine. Regardless of the pathogenesis, the symptoms of anaphylaxis are identical.

EPIDEMIOLOGY, MORBIDITIES, AND MORTALITIES

The lifetime risk of anaphylaxis is at least 1.6% in the general population in the United States.[5,6] The hospital admission rate for anaphylaxis in the United States for both children and adults had increased from 2000 to 2011.[5] Children between 0 and 4 years of age are at the highest risk for hospitalization because of anaphylaxis, with the main cause being food allergy.[5]

Overall fatality rates from anaphylaxis remain stable at 0.63 to 0.76 per million US adults per year.[5,7] This prevalence is higher than that reported from the United Kingdom (0.33 per million),[8] similar to the rate reported from Australia (0.64 per million),[9] but lower than that reported from France (0.83 per million).[10] In the United States, the most common causes of anaphylaxis fatalities in adults are medications (58.8%), followed by unspecified causes (19.3%), venoms (15.2%), and foods (6.7%).[7] Fatal anaphylaxis is significantly associated with African American ethnicity and older age.[7] However, fatal anaphylaxis caused by venom is more common in white people.[7]

Data about fatal anaphylaxis in the pediatric population are insufficient and variable from country to country.[11–13] For example, in the United States and Australia, medications were found to be the most common cause of pediatric fatalities caused by anaphylaxis. However, a study from the United Kingdom identified foods as the most common cause of fatal anaphylaxis in patients less than 30 years of age. Factors associated with a higher risk for fatal food-induced anaphylaxis include adolescent age, history of a reaction, allergy to peanuts or tree nuts, asthma, and the absence of cutaneous symptoms.[1]

CAUSES
Food

Food allergy is the most common cause of anaphylaxis. The most common foods causing anaphylaxis are cow's milk (infants), peanuts (children), and tree nuts and shellfish (young adults).[1,2,5] Rare, delayed anaphylaxis occurring several hours after eating mammalian red meat are widely reported caused by IgE antibodies against the carbohydrate structure galactose-alpha-1,3-galactose. This reaction has been linked to sensitization from multiple tick bites.[1,5]

Drugs

Drugs are the second most common cause of anaphylaxis. The most common culprit of medication-induced anaphylaxis is beta-lactam antibiotics, followed by nonsteroidal antiinflammatory drugs (NSAIDs).

Reactions to vancomycin, known as red man syndrome or red neck syndrome, can mimic anaphylaxis. These reactions are non–IgE mediated, caused by direct mast cell activation, and can therefore occur with the first administration of vancomycin. Such reactions are preventable by slowing the infusion rate and premedicating with antihistamines.

Radiocontrast media reactions are also caused by direct mast cell activation and/or activation of coagulation/complement cascades. The use of lower osmolality preparations and premedication with steroid and antihistamines is recommended to minimize its occurrence.

Multiple agents may be involved in perioperative anaphylaxis, including antibiotics, neuromuscular blocking agents, blood products, chlorhexidine, and natural rubber latex.[1,5] Detailed clinical investigation may elucidate the cause of perioperative anaphylaxis.

Latex

Incidence of latex-induced anaphylaxis in the United States has stabilized because of the use of nonlatex products in hospitals and clinics, although latex allergy remains an important cause of anaphylaxis outside the United States.[5]

Hymenoptera

Another important cause of anaphylaxis is insect sting hypersensitivity reaction. The culprit insects include flying hymenopterans (yellow jacket, hornet, wasp, honeybee) and imported fire ant.[14]

Exercise-induced Anaphylaxis

Exercise-induced anaphylaxis (EIA) occurs after physical exertion and can be a difficult diagnosis. Direct mast cell activation is thought to play role in EIA. Some EIA can be related to certain foods, particularly wheat. A supervised exercise challenge test is not helpful in all cases. Avoiding exercise in the immediate postprandial period, exercising with a partner, prompt recognition of anaphylactic symptoms, and self-use of epinephrine autoinjectors are recommended.[1]

Idiopathic

Idiopathic anaphylaxis is a diagnosis of exclusion. Idiopathic anaphylaxis in children is very rare. In contrast, the cause of anaphylaxis in adults may remain undetermined in up to two-thirds of the cases when evaluated by specialists per survey studies.[2] Important considerations should include mast cell disorders and mastocytosis for these patients.

Causes of anaphylaxis are summarized in **Table 1**.[1,2,5]

Signs and Symptoms

The most common clinical findings in anaphylaxis involve the skin/mucosa (62%–90%), followed by respiratory (45%–70%) and gastrointestinal symptoms (25%–45%).[2,3] Urticaria, pruritus, and angioedema are among the common skin/mucosal presentations of anaphylaxis. Angioedema may involve eyelids, conjunctiva, lips, tongue, uvula, and oral pharyngeal mucosa. In some cases, pruritus can be seen alone without evidence of hives or urticaria on physical examination.[2]

Table 1
Common causes of anaphylaxis

Pathophysiology of Anaphylaxis	Common Causes
Classic IgE-mediated anaphylaxis	Food (milk, egg, peanuts, tree nuts, seafood, soy, wheat), drug (antibiotics, NSAIDs, biologic agents, neuromuscular blocking agents, barbiturates), latex, insect sting, subcutaneous allergen immunotherapy, seminal fluid
Immune complex complement-related anaphylaxis	Blood products, hemodialysis
Nonimmunologic anaphylaxis	RCM, opioids, ethanol, physical exercise, cold, heat, sunlight/UV radiation
Idiopathic anaphylaxis	Unknown

Abbreviations: RCM, radiocontrast media; UV, ultraviolet.
Data from Refs.[1,2,5]

Upper airway obstruction, wheezing, and/or hypoxia are frequently seen in anaphylaxis and can be life threatening. Abdominal pain, nausea, vomiting, and/or diarrhea are also commonly observed. Notably, 10% of the patients can present with immediate, profound shock without cutaneous involvement, making the diagnosis of anaphylaxis more challenging.[2,3] Clinical features of anaphylaxis are summarized in **Table 2**.[2,3]

Biphasic anaphylaxis is reported in 0.4% to 23.3% of patients with anaphylaxis.[1,5] It is described as a second anaphylactic reaction that occurs within 12 hours after the resolution of the initial anaphylaxis and without new exposure to allergens. Protracted anaphylaxis is an anaphylactic reaction that can last from hours to several days without resolution of symptoms.

It is important to distinguish and identify clinical mimickers of anaphylaxis as listed in **Table 3**.[1]

DIAGNOSIS

The diagnosis of anaphylaxis is often challenging and missed, compromising the well-being of patients. The diagnosis of anaphylaxis should be considered in the following 3 situations:

Table 2
Common signs and symptoms of anaphylaxis by organ systems

Organ System Involvement	Presentations
Skin/mucosa (62%–90%)	Pruritus with or without rash, urticaria, flushing, angioedema of the lips/tongue and/or uvula, conjunctival edema, periorbital edema
Respiratory (45%–70%)	Nasal congestion, rhinitis, dyspnea, stridor, sensation of throat closing, choking, wheezing, hypoxia
Gastrointestinal (25%–45%)	Nausea, vomiting, diarrhea, abdominal pain
Cardiovascular (10%–45%)	Diaphoresis, chest pain, presyncope/syncope, tachycardia, bradycardia (caused by Bezold-Jarisch reflex), hypotension, end-organ dysfunction
Central nervous system (5%–15%)	Confusion, unconsciousness, hypotonia, headache, incontinence, seizure

Data from Adkinson NF Jr. BB, Busse WW, Holgate ST, Lemanske RF Jr., Simons FER and Middleton's Allergy: Principles and Practice. 7th ed. St. Louis: Mosby, Inc; 2009 and Simons FE. Anaphylaxis, killer allergy: long-term management in the community. Allergy Clin Immunol. 2006;117(2):367-377.

Table 3
Differential diagnosis of anaphylaxis

Differential Diagnosis	Distinguish Clinical Features
Flushing syndromes	
Drug/ingestant induced	Flushing with history of exposure to alcohol, ACE inhibitors, niacin, nicotine, or catecholamines
Pheochromocytoma	Flushing, headaches, diaphoresis, tachycardia, with hypertension. Increased neuropeptide levels
Carcinoid tumor/vasointestinal polypeptide tumors	Flushing with secretory diarrhea, abdominal pain, diaphoresis, bronchospasm, and tremor. Increased neuropeptide levels
Medullary carcinoma of the thyroid	Facial/upper-extremity flushing, telangiectasias, thyroid nodules Increased serum calcitonin and CEA levels
Mastocytosis and mast cell activating syndrome	Symptoms mimic those of anaphylaxis Typically recurrent. May have urticaria pigmentosa; positive Darier sign is supportive for the diagnosis. Need further laboratory tests to help diagnosis (see **Table 4**)
Vasodepressor reactions or vasovagal reactions	Hypotension, weakness, pallor, diaphoresis, nausea, vomiting, and bradycardia without cutaneous manifestations
Restaurant syndromes	
Monosodium glutamate	Flushing with headache, nausea, diaphoresis, numbness, or burning in the mouth/throat. Typically after exposure to food from Chinese restaurant
Scombroidosis	History of exposure to spoiled, scombroid fish (tunas, mackerels, bonitos). More than 1 person with symptoms. Skin finding is flushing (sunburnlike) rather than urticaria. Normal serum tryptase level
Nonorganic disease	
Panic attacks	Sudden periods of intense fear, palpitations, diaphoresis, shortness of breath, numbness without cutaneous findings except for possible mild flushing
VCD	Throat tightness, dyspnea, dysphonia, stridor, wheezing, coughing, without cutaneous findings Pulmonary function test showed extrathoracic airway obstruction of flattening of the inspiratory flow volume loop. Flexible laryngoscopy showed abnormal adduction of vocal cords
Munchausen stridor (factitious anaphylaxis)	Symptoms of vocal cord dysfunction. Patients consciously produce symptoms of illness for secondary gain
Undifferentiated somatoform anaphylaxis	Symptoms of dyspnea, throat tightness, syncope without physical findings of wheezing, hypotension, or cutaneous manifestations
Miscellaneous	
HAE accompanied by rash	History of recurrent episodes of angioedema without pruritus that are commonly self-limited and resolve within 2–5 d without treatment. A family history of angioedema is helpful for the diagnosis

(continued on next page)

Table 3 (continued)	
Differential Diagnosis	**Distinguish Clinical Features**
Red man syndrome	History of vancomycin administration with symptoms of flushing and pruritus on the face, neck, and upper body. Hypotension is possible
Capillary leak syndrome	Recurrent angioedema, gastrointestinal symptoms, shock with hemoconcentration, usually associated with monoclonal gammopathy

Abbreviations: ACE, angiotensin-converting enzyme; CEA, carcinoembryonic antigen; HAE, hereditary angioedema; VCD, vocal cord dysfunction.

Data from Lieberman P, Nicklas RA, Randolph C, et al. Anaphylaxis–a practice parameter update 2015. Ann Allergy Asthma Immunol. 2015;115(5):341-384.

1. Patients who experience acute onset and rapidly progressive symptoms (minutes to hours) involving the skin and/or mucous membranes plus either respiratory symptoms or hypotension/end-organ dysfunction.
2. Patients who experience acute onset of symptoms (minutes to hours) after exposure to a likely allergen and have at least 2 organ systems involved.
3. Patients who experience an acute decrease in blood pressure (minutes to hour) after exposure to a known allergen, even without other symptoms.

LABORATORY FINDINGS

Anaphylaxis is essentially a clinical diagnosis and most laboratory tests are not commonly required.[1,5]

Serum histamine levels decrease to the baseline within an hour after the onset of anaphylaxis and are unlikely to be helpful.[1] However, serum tryptase can be useful for confirming the diagnosis of anaphylaxis, especially in cases of clinically ambiguous presentations. Serum tryptase levels remain increased for up to 6 hours after the onset of anaphylaxis[1] and could theoretically be obtained in the emergency department (ED) if needed.

Persistent increase of serum tryptase level for more than 24 hours after the resolution of anaphylaxis indicates underlying mast cell disorders and mastocytosis.[1] These patients can present with recurrent idiopathic anaphylaxis. Further laboratory evaluation and a referral to a specialist are recommended.

Other laboratory tests that are helpful for identifying the cause of anaphylaxis include skin prick testing and allergen-specific serum IgE levels. Because of high sensitivity and lower specificity, skin prick testing and allergen-specific serum IgE levels should focus only on suspected allergen exposure suggested by history.[1,2,15] Testing with broad allergen panels is not recommended and can lead to false-positive tests and unnecessary allergen avoidance, especially food.[15] A referral to a specialist should be considered to identify the cause of anaphylaxis. Typically, skin prick testing is delayed for 6 weeks after anaphylaxis because of the possibility of specific IgE consumption that occurred during the reaction; however, the evidence supporting this practice is controversial.

Table 4 summarizes laboratory tests that may be useful for diagnosis and in identifying the cause of anaphylaxis.[1,2,15]

MANAGEMENT
Acute Management of Anaphylaxis

Epinephrine at 0.01 mg/kg (maximum dose of 0.5 mg) per single dose is the first drug of choice for treating anaphylaxis. There are no absolute contraindications to

Table 4	
Laboratory tests for the diagnosis or establishing the cause of anaphylaxis	
Test	**Features/Usage**
Histamine	Serum histamine level is increased 2–15 min after the onset of anaphylaxis and decreased to baseline by 1 h. This short period of detection makes serum histamine not practical for diagnosis of anaphylaxis in clinical settings
	However, urine histamine can be helpful for the diagnosis of anaphylaxis. This test is practically challenging because it requires a standard 24-h urine collection and, ideally, a second baseline sample 24 h after the resolution of anaphylaxis
Tryptase	Serum tryptase level peaks at 60–90 min after the onset of anaphylaxis and remains increased up to 6 h. This test can be useful for confirming the diagnosis of anaphylaxis, although it may not be increased in food-induced anaphylaxis
	If serum tryptase remains increased 24 h after the resolution of anaphylaxis, further tests for mastocytosis and mast cell activation syndrome should be entertained (discussed in the text in relation to bone marrow biopsy)
	Patients who experienced insect sting anaphylaxis should have baseline serum tryptase tested because of high risk of having occult systemic mastocytosis
	Serum tryptase level is also increased in nonanaphylaxis conditions such as acute myelocytic leukemia, myelodysplastic syndromes, acquired C1 esterase deficiency in non-Hodgkin lymphoma, hypereosinophilic syndrome associated with the FIP1 L1-PDGFRA mutation, and end-stage renal disease with increased levels of endogenous stem cell factor
Skin and in vitro tests for serum-specific IgE	Useful for determining the cause of anaphylaxis for suspicious food or drug allergens
	For food-induced anaphylaxis, these tests should be focused on foods suspected of provoking the reaction. Fresh food prick skin test may be needed in cases of fruit or vegetable allergy, or when extracts for foods are not available
	Oral food challenge may be needed if the diagnosis of food anaphylaxis remains unclear
Bone marrow aspiration/ biopsy and mutational analysis of KIT showing a codon 816 mutation (Asp816Val)	Useful for confirming the diagnosis of mast cell disorders as a differential diagnosis of anaphylaxis
	Bone marrow specimen showed coexpression of CD2 and CD25 in CD117 (KIT)-positive mast cells by flow cytometry

Abbreviation: CD, cluster of differentiation.
Data from Refs.[1,2,15]

epinephrine. Transient side effects of epinephrine, such as pallor, tremor, palpitations, anxiety, headache, and dizziness, are common with the therapeutic doses and generally not cause for concern.[3,16] Delayed epinephrine injection increases the risk of hospitalization and death from anaphylaxis.[5]

Prompt recognition of anaphylaxis and early administration of epinephrine, even before the ED arrival, are strongly encouraged. Epinephrine should be administered intramuscularly in the midouter thigh or intravenously if intravenous access is readily available. Subcutaneous injection is discouraged because of poor circulation to subcutaneous tissue in anaphylaxis. Epinephrine can be repeated up to 3 times every 5 to 15 minutes if the patient is not clinically responding.

After epinephrine administration, the patient should be removed from the inciting allergen if exposure continues to occur; for example, discontinuing infusion of a medication or removing the patient from the nesting area of stinging insects. Cardiopulmonary resuscitation; assessment of airway, breathing, circulation; and activation of the emergency medical services should be initiated.[1] Adults and adolescents should be placed in a recumbent position. Young children should be placed in a comfort position, and pregnant women should be placed on the left side. Supplemental oxygen should also be initiated. Intravenous access and fluid replacement for hypotension should be started as soon as possible. Intraosseous access can be considered if intravenous access is not readily available.

Nebulized albuterol should be considered in patients with lower airway obstruction and can be repeated every 15 minutes, if required. Glucagon should be administered in patient on β-blockers who do not respond to epinephrine. Advanced airway management may be needed in patients with severe stridor or laryngeal edema. Consider dopamine infusion, in addition to epinephrine infusion, in patients with refractory hypotension caused by anaphylaxis.[1]

H1 and H2 antihistamines and corticosteroids are considered as optional or adjunctive medications for anaphylaxis. These medications are not lifesaving and should not be given as monotherapy or the initial treatment of anaphylaxis.[5] First-generation and second-generation H1 antihistamines have a delayed onset of action and do not stop mast cell degranulation. Although they can relieve dermatologic symptoms, including urticaria, H1 antihistamines cannot relieve the hypotension or airway obstruction caused by anaphylaxis and hence should not replace epinephrine. Because they are to be considered only as adjunctive therapies, there are no well-designed, randomized, placebo-controlled trials establishing the use of H2 antihistamines in the treatment of anaphylaxis.[1,5]

Glucocorticoids also have no role in the initial treatment of anaphylaxis. In addition to a slow onset of action, their use and dosage in anaphylaxis are extrapolated from studies on acute asthma. The use of steroids for preventing biphasic or protracted anaphylaxis is also not strongly supported in many studies.[1,5,17,18]

At least 4 to 8 hours of direct observation and monitoring is recommended for moderate to severe anaphylaxis. A longer observation should be considered in patients who are at risk of severe anaphylaxis (eg, asthmatics, medical comorbidities, requiring more than 1 dose of epinephrine, prolonged symptoms of anaphylaxis, exposure to ingested allergens, or pharyngeal edema). Biphasic anaphylaxis occurs in between 0.4% and 23.3% of anaphylaxis episodes and usually occurs in patients presenting with hypotension or with unknown triggers. Therefore, routine prolonged monitoring is no longer necessary in patients whose anaphylaxis symptoms have resolved. However, patients and caregivers should be provided with and instructed in the use of epinephrine autoinjectors and educated to recognize anaphylaxis on all hospital discharges.[1,5]

Long-term Management of Anaphylaxis

Self-treatment: autoinjectable epinephrine and emergency action plan for anaphylaxis
Autoinjectable epinephrine should be prescribed to all patients who have experienced anaphylaxis or those who are at risk for anaphylaxis. At least 2 epinephrine autoinjectors should be given because up to 30% of anaphylactic patients require the second dose of epinephrine.[1] Historically, 2 doses of the epinephrine autoinjectors have been available in the United States: 0.15 mg (for patient weights of <30 kg) and 0.3 mg (for patient weights of ≥30 kg). In early 2018, a new 0.1-mg dose of the epinephrine autoinjector was made available for children weighing 7.5 to 15 kg. As stated earlier, the

recommended dose for epinephrine in anaphylaxis is 0.01 mg/kg, with a maximum single dose of 0.5 mg. Therefore, a single 0.3-mg dose may be suboptimal in teens as well as obese children, requiring repeat injection of epinephrine. In addition, the needle length of the autoinjectors may be too short to reach the thigh muscles in obese patients.[16] Given the safety profile of epinephrine and the potential for subtherapeutic treatment, providers should consider choosing a slightly higher dose for some patients.[1]

The most significant obstacle for long-term management of anaphylaxis is the underprescription and underuse of epinephrine. Available epinephrine autoinjectors vary in size, shape, color, needle size, method of use, ease of use, and portability.[5,16] Health care providers should be familiar with the device prescribed and able to instruct patients and parents in its use. Epinephrine autoinjectors should be kept at 20°C to 25°C to protect against degradation of the medication and ensure the mechanical integrity of the devices. Higher temperatures can increase the degradation of epinephrine. Exposure to freezing temperatures for a few days does not cause medication degradation but the device should be completely thawed before use.[5]

Personalized emergency action plans should be provided to all patients at risk for anaphylaxis (available at the American Academy of Allergy, Asthma, and Immunology Web site, www.aaaai.org). Plans should include common signs and symptoms of anaphylaxis, instructions for epinephrine autoinjector use, and contact information for emergency medical services for transportation to an ED.[15] Patients at risk for anaphylaxis should also wear medical identification listing their anaphylactic triggers, comorbidities, and concurrent medications. Such identification could be in the form of Medic-Alert jewelry or an anaphylaxis wallet card (also available at www.aaaai.org).[1,16]

Prevention of recurrence of anaphylaxis and specialist referral

A referral to an allergist/immunologist should be considered in all patients who have experienced anaphylaxis. Specialist referrals have shown improved clinical outcomes and reduced hospital admissions caused by early diagnosis in addition to identification of anaphylaxis-inducing allergens. Regular follow-up of such patients also showed long-term risk reduction of anaphylaxis.[1,5] All patients and caregivers should be provided with written and specific information on avoidance of known allergens. Personalized emergency action plans should be reviewed periodically at follow-up visits.[3,5,16]

Food Avoidance of culprit food allergens remains the mainstay of treatment of food-induced anaphylaxis. Patients and caregivers should be educated on how to read and interpret product ingredient labels, inquire about allergen exposure at restaurants, as well as avoid cross-contamination and eating cross-reactive foods.[1,3,5,16] Evaluation by an allergist, including skin prick testing, food allergen component testing, or oral food challenge, can help confirm the cause of anaphylaxis and also determine whether patients have outgrown their sensitivity, particularly to milk or egg. In cases of multiple dietary restrictions, a referral to a nutritionist should be considered. Desensitization by oral or sublingual immunotherapy has been achieved in multiple randomized controlled research trials but has not yet been approved for clinical use.[1,5,16]

Exclusive breastfeeding is recommended for the first 4 to 6 months of life. Specific food allergen avoidance by mothers during pregnancy or breastfeeding has not proved effective for primary prevention of food allergies.[15] Introduction of solid foods, including common allergenic foods, should not be delayed beyond 6 months of age. In children at high risk for food allergies (eg, children with early development of severe atopic disease or whose parent or sibling has confirmed peanut allergy), specific IgE testing (serum or skin prick testing) for milk, egg, and peanut can be considered before the introduction of these highly allergenic foods. The widespread use of specific IgE testing in children who are not at high risk for food allergy is not recommended because such testing can lead to unnecessary dietary restrictions.[15]

Drug Patients with drug-induced anaphylaxis should strictly avoid the culprit medication. They also should be educated regarding other drug therapies that might cross-react. An alternative, non–cross-reacting medication from a different class should be offered, if possible. An allergist consultation for a desensitization procedure may be needed if the anaphylaxis-inducing medication cannot be avoided. An outpatient referral to an allergist can also aid in confirmation of drug allergy by means of skin prick testing, intradermal testing, and/or graded challenge of the medication, particularly in patients with penicillin allergy.[3,5,16]

Hymenoptera Patients with insect-induced anaphylaxis should be educated on measures to avoid insect stings. They should be referred to an allergist for considerations of venom testing and immunotherapy because immunotherapy can significantly reduce the risk of recurrent severe systemic reaction on subsequent stings.[5,14] Hymenoptera venom and whole-body extract (fire ant) skin testing and venom immunotherapy are recommended for all patients with anaphylaxis or patients greater than or equal to 16 years old with cutaneous systemic reaction because of high risk of anaphylaxis with subsequent sting in these patients. In contrast, venom testing or immunotherapy is not indicated for children younger than 16 years of age who have cutaneous systemic reaction, or for patients who developed only large local reactions because of the low risk of anaphylaxis with subsequent stings.[14]

SUMMARY

Anaphylaxis is a life-threatening reaction that should be recognized promptly. The most common causes of anaphylaxis are foods and medications. Common symptoms of anaphylaxis include urticaria, angioedema, respiratory distress, nausea, vomiting, diarrhea, and hypotension. The symptoms can occur within minutes to hours after allergen exposure. Up to 10% of patients with anaphylaxis can present without cutaneous findings. This lack of skin/mucosal involvement can lead to misdiagnosis or delayed diagnosis of anaphylaxis. Epinephrine is the drug of choice for treating anaphylaxis. The most significant obstacle for long-term management of anaphylaxis is the underprescription and underuse of epinephrine. Delayed epinephrine administration in anaphylaxis is associated with increase in morbidity and mortality. At least 2 epinephrine autoinjectors should be prescribed because up to 30% of anaphylactic patients require the second dose of epinephrine. Patients and caregivers should be educated on the use of epinephrine autoinjectors with periodic review of symptoms and emergency action plan for anaphylaxis. A referral to an allergist/immunologist should be considered in all patients who have experienced anaphylaxis. Specialist referrals have shown improved clinical outcomes and reduced hospital admissions caused by early diagnosis in addition to identification of anaphylaxis-inducing allergens.

REFERENCES

1. Lieberman P, Nicklas RA, Randolph C, et al. Anaphylaxis–a practice parameter update 2015. Ann Allergy Asthma Immunol 2015;115(5):341–84.

2. Adkinson NF Jr, Bochner BS, Busse WW, et al. Middleton's allergy: principles and practice. 7th edition. St Louis (MO): Mosby, Inc; 2009.

3. Simons FE. Anaphylaxis, killer allergy: long-term management in the community. Allergy Clin Immunol 2006;117(2):367–77.

4. Sampson HA, Munoz-Furlong A, Campbell RL, et al. Second symposium on the definition and management of anaphylaxis: summary report–second National Institute of Allergy and Infectious Disease/Food Allergy and Anaphylaxis Network symposium. Ann Emerg Med 2006;47(4):373–80.

5. Simons FE, Ebisawa M, Sanchez-Borges M, et al. 2015 update of the evidence base: World Allergy Organization anaphylaxis guidelines. World Allergy Organ J 2015;8(1):32.

6. Wood RA, Camargo CA Jr, Lieberman P, et al. Anaphylaxis in America: the prevalence and characteristics of anaphylaxis in the United States. J Allergy Clin Immunol 2014;133:461–7.

7. Jerschow E, Lin RY, Scaperotti MM, et al. Fatal anaphylaxis in the United States, 1999–2010: temporal patterns and demographic associations. J Allergy Clin Immunol 2014;134:1318–28.e7.

8. Pumphrey R. Anaphylaxis: can we tell who is at risk of a fatal reaction? Curr Opin Allergy Clin Immunol 2004;4:285–90.

9. Liew WK, Williamson E, Tang ML. Anaphylaxis fatalities and admissions in Australia. J Allergy Clin Immunol 2009;123:434–42.

10. Pouessel G, Claverie C, Labreuche J, et al. Fatal anaphylaxis in France: analysis of national anaphylaxis data, 1979- 2011. J Allergy Clin Immunol 2017;140:610–2.

11. Ma L, Danoff TM, Borish L. Case fatality and population mortality associated with anaphylaxis in the United States. J Allergy Clin Immunol 2014;133:1075–83.

12. Turner PJ, Gowland MH, Sharma V, et al. Increase in anaphylaxis- related hospitalizations but no increase in fatalities: an analysis of United Kingdom national anaphylaxis data, 1992-2012. J Allergy Clin Immunol 2015;135:956–63.

13. Mullins RJ, Wainstein BK, Barnes EH, et al. Increases in anaphylaxis fatalities in Australia from 1997 to 2013. Clin Exp Allergy 2016;46:1099–110.

14. Golden DB, Demain J, Freeman T, et al. Stinging insect hypersensitivity: a practice parameter update 2016. Ann Allergy Asthma Immunol 2017;118(1):28–54.

15. Sampson HA, Aceves S, Bock SA, et al. Food allergy: a practice parameter update-2014. J Allergy Clin Immunol 2014;134(5):1016–25.e43.

16. Simons FE. Anaphylaxis: recent advances in assessment and treatment. J Allergy Clin Immunol 2009;124(4):625–36.

17. Lieberman P. Biphasic anaphylactic reactions. Ann Allergy Asthma Immunol 2005;95(3):217–26.

18. Choo KJ, Simons E, Sheikh A. Glucocorticoids for the treatment of anaphylaxis: cochrane systematic review. Allergy 2010;65(10):1205–11.

Biologic Agents and Secondary Immune Deficiency

Heather Axelrod, MD[a], Matthew Adams, MD[b],*

KEYWORDS

- Secondary immune deficiency • Biologics • Immunosuppression
- Monoclonal antibodies • TNF-α inhibitors • Anti-inflammatory

KEY POINTS

- Biologics are protein-based pharmaceuticals derived from living organisms or their products, and are widely used in treatment of autoimmune and autoinflammatory diseases.
- The use of biologics has become the standard of care for many pediatric rheumatologic conditions because of their efficacy in disease remission.
- TNF-α inhibitors are the oldest and best studied with regard to immune suppression and possible infectious consequences.
- Pediatricians need to be aware of immune suppression caused by biologics and the spectrum of infections that should be screened for before use (especially TB) and during use.
- Specific guidelines for screening, measures to reduce risk, and precautions to be given to patients on biologics do not yet exist for children, and are needed.

Biologics block inflammatory pathways, which reduce pathologic inflammation through various mechanisms including cytokine inhibition, nonclonal cell deletion, and co-stimulatory inhibition. It is not surprising that this immune suppression raises concern for secondary immunodeficiency and increased risk of infection. Clinical studies by Keyser,[1] Rutherford and colleagues,[2] Bradshaw and colleagues,[3] Carneiro and colleagues,[4] and Lee and colleagues[5] have investigated and detailed the association of these therapies with opportunistic infections and malignancies.

Biologics are classified by their mode of action. The first biologic developed and approved for the treatment of rheumatoid arthritis (RA) was the tumor necrosis factor alpha (TNF-α) inhibitor etanercept. Other subsequent TNF-α inhibitors include

Conflict of Interest: The authors declare no relevant conflict of interest.
[a] Department of Pediatrics (PGY3), Children's Hospital of Michigan, Detroit, MI, USA; [b] Division of Pediatric Rheumatology, Department of Pediatrics, Children's Hospital of Michigan, Wayne State University, 3950 Beaubien Boulevard, Detroit, MI 48201, USA
* Corresponding author.
E-mail address: madams3@dmc.org

certolizumab, adalimumab, infliximab, and golimumab. Other classes of biologics include B cell inhibitors (rituximab), interleukin 1 (IL-1) inhibitors (anakinra), IL-6 inhibitors (sarilumab and tocilizumab [TCZ]), and cytotoxic T lymphocyte-associated antigen 4 (CTLA4) co-stimulator inhibitors (abatacept/Orencia).

We discuss the mechanism of action of the currently approved biologics and summarize the studies on immune suppression from biologics, most of which have been conducted patients with rheumatology.

TUMOR NECROSIS FACTOR ALPHA INHIBITORS

TNF-α is a cytokine that modulates the host response in the acute phase of infection and induces production of IL-1, IL-2, IL-6, IL-8, monocyte chemoattractant protein-1, gas chromatography-mass spectrometry, and adhesion molecules such as E-selectin and vascular cell adhesion molecule 1.[6] TNF-α inhibitors remove TNF-α from the extracellular environment. They have been shown to be effective in treating RA, juvenile idiopathic arthritis (JIA), inflammatory bowel disease, and the spondyloarthropathies. By inhibiting TNF-α, these biologic agents also inhibit the initiation of an inflammatory response and may leave the body susceptible to infection. Furthermore, the diagnosis of a bacterial infection may not be made as quickly because of the lack of certain clinical features (ie, fever or elevated C-reactive protein). The association between TNF-α inhibitors and infection has been well established in the literature, and in 2011 a black box warning was issued to warn providers and adult patients about the risk of serious infections when using these products.

Etanercept is a dimeric fusion protein with 2 TNF-α receptors linked to the Fc portion of human immunoglobulin G1 (IgG1). It was the first anti-TNF agent to be approved by the Food and Drug Administration (FDA) for the treatment of RA. Over the past 16 years, its short-term safety profile has been investigated in many clinical trials in patients with RA, psoriatic arthritis, and psoriasis.[7–10] There are 2 major clinical trials that looked at the use of etanercept in RA; the TEMPO[11] and COMET studies.[12]

The TEMPO study, published in February 2004, included 522 patients. The percentage of serious infection (not defined in the study) was 4% in all groups: those receiving methotrexate (MTX) alone, those receiving a combination of etanercept and MTX, and those receiving etanercept monotherapy. This study did not identify the infections that developed. Six malignant diseases were noted. One patient in each group had basal cell carcinoma, and there was 1 case of breast cancer, melanoma, and rectal cancer in the etanercept group. There were no cases of central demyelinating diseases, blood dyscrasias, or multiple sclerosis.

The COMET study, published in August 2008, examined 2 groups; an MTX monotherapy group and a combined treatment group receiving etanercept and MTX. Almost 92% of patients in the MTX group and 90% in the combined group reported an adverse event. The most common adverse events were nausea and nasopharyngitis. Serious adverse events (SAEs) occurred in 12.7% of patients in the MTX-only group and 12% of patients in the combined group. The most common SAEs included worsening of RA, breast cancer, chest pain, pneumonia, cholelithiasis, interstitial lung disease, disc protrusion, and hip arthroplasty. One patient died of acute respiratory failure. Eight patients in the MTX group and 5 in the combined group developed serious infections. Herpes zoster was seen in 1 patient in the MTX group. There were no cases of tuberculosis (TB) or demyelinating diseases. There were 8 malignant diseases reported. None of these were found to be related to MTX or etanercept.

The TEMPO and COMET studies demonstrated that etanercept is generally well tolerated in RA, but SAEs are still evident. In the British Society for Rheumatology

Biologics Registry for Rheumatoid Arthritis prospective observational study in 2001, etanercept was shown to have the lowest incidence of TB compared with the other TNF-α inhibitors.[13] A similar result was seen in a study in 2009, which demonstrated that etanercept had a lower risk of causing reactivation TB than infliximab or adalimumab.[14] In a long-term clinical trial over 8 years of patients on etanercept, the safety profile was shown to be similar to that seen in studies over a shorter time frame.[15] Registries continue to assess long-term risk and harm of etanercept in patients with rheumatologic conditions.[16]

Adalimumab is a human monoclonal antibody that blocks the effects of TNF-α. Adalimumab was the first therapeutic monoclonal antibody against TNF-α that had 100% human peptide sequences and is thereby indistinguishable in function and structure from human IgG1.[17] There were 4 randomized double-blinded placebo-controlled clinical trials were used for the original application of this medication: the ARMADA,[18] DE019,[19] DE011,[20] and STAR studies.[21]

The ARMADA study, published in January 2003, examined a group of patients taking adalimumab and MTX or MTX with a placebo over 24 weeks. Infections occurred at a similar rate in the patients treated with adalimumab (1.55/patient-year) and those treated with a placebo (1.38/patient-year). Two patients in the adalimumab group developed pneumonia and remained in the study. One patient in the treatment group developed adenocarcinoma of the colon. No other cancers were reported, no drug-related toxicity occurred, and no patients developed TB or lupus-like syndrome.

In the DE019 study, published in May 2004, adalimumab was used alone at a dosage of 20 mg once a week, or 40 mg every other week with MTX, in 618 patients over 52 weeks.

The rate of SAEs was 14.3%. More patients (3.8%) treated with adalimumab reported serious infections requiring hospitalization compared with the placebo group (0.5%). There was a statistically significant difference between the percentage of patients reporting serious infections who received adalimumab 40 mg every other week and the placebo group. However, there was no statistically significant difference between the rates of serious infections in the group that received adalimumab weekly and the placebo group. On entry, 2.6% of patients receiving adalimumab and 3.5% of patients receiving placebo were positive for purified protein derivative (PPD).

One patient in the treatment group receiving adalimumab 40 mg every other week was diagnosed with primary TB, withdrew from the study, and was treated. Before the start of the study this patient had a normal chest radiograph and was negative for PPD.

One patient in the group that received 40 mg adalimumab every other week developed a histoplasmosis infection. Another patient in the 40-mg group developed herpes zoster and encephalitis. Four patients receiving adalimumab developed cancers; non-Hodgkin lymphoma, adenocarcinoma, breast cancer, and testicular seminoma, respectively. One patient in the 20-mg treatment group had worsening of a central demyelinating illness. There were 2 deaths in the 40-mg treatment group, 1 attributed to urosepsis and 1 from multiple fractures. There was 1 death in the 20-mg treatment group related to complications of chemotherapy for the treatment of lymphoma. No deaths occurred in the placebo group.

The DE011 study, published in May 2004, investigated adalimumab as monotherapy at varying dosages and frequency of treatment. Over 26 weeks, 544 patients with RA were separated into groups receiving adalimumab: 20 mg every other week, 20 mg weekly, 40 mg every other week, 40 mg weekly, or a placebo. Adalimumab was well tolerated, and most adverse events were mild or moderately severe. The rate of adverse events was 2.23 patients/patient-year in the adalimumab-treated group and 2.60 patients/patient-year in the placebo group. There was no statistically significant difference in the rates of SAEs between the placebo group and the adalimumab-treated group (0% and 2.3% of patients, respectively). In addition, there were no dose-related statistically significant adverse events for those in the adalimumab group. There were no cases of TB. There was an equal rate of malignancies between the treatment and placebo group, and they were deemed to be unrelated to the study drug.

The STAR study, published in December 2003, investigated adalimumab in combination with several anti-RA drugs, including methotrexate, sulfasalazine, hydroxychloroquine, leflunomide, and prednisolone, sometimes with more than 1 of these drugs being used with adalimumab, as opposed to disease-modifying antirheumatic drugs (DMARDS—a category of drugs defined by their use in rheumatologic disease rather than by their mode of action) and a placebo. The study included 318 patients over 24 weeks and found no statistically significant differences in SAEs, or severe or life-threatening adverse events leading to withdrawal between the adalimumab plus DMARDs group and the placebo plus DMARDs group.

Infliximab (Remicade), is a chimeric human and mouse peptide sequence monoclonal antibody to TNF-α. The ASPIRE[22] and BeST[23] trials investigated the safety and efficacy of infliximab in patients with early RA. The ATTRACT[24] study examined patients with an established history of 7 to 9 years of RA taking infliximab.

The ATTRACT study, published in November 30, 2000, included 428 patients with established RA of 7.2 to 9 years in duration which persisted despite treatment with MTX for 3 months or longer. There were 2 treatment groups, those that received MTX alone and those that received infliximab and MTX. SAEs occurred in 21% of MTX group and 17% in the infliximab and MTX group. The frequency of serious infections was also similar (8% and 6%, respectively, of the MTX and infliximab plus MTX groups). The most common adverse events were upper respiratory tract infections, pharyngitis, sinusitis, and headache. Five patients receiving infliximab developed cancer; basal cell carcinoma, and rectal carcinoma. Eight deaths occurred during the trial, 3% in the MTX-only group and 1% in the infliximab plus MTX group.

The ASPIRE trial, published in November 2004, examined the efficacy of infliximab in over 1000 patients with early moderate to severely active RA. These patients were examined over a 54-week period. SAEs were more prevalent in the MTX-infliximab group than the MTX-placebo group; the rates were 14% and 11%, respectively. Pneumonia occurred more frequently in those treated with infliximab than those with MTX alone. Most of the 15 cases (or 2%) in the infliximab group were community acquired pneumonias. Active TB was diagnosed in 4 patients from the infliximab treatment groups. Three of the 4 had pulmonary TB. Four patients in the infliximab group were diagnosed with a malignancy during the trial. Four patients died during the study, 2 were from the group treated with infliximab. None of the deaths were thought to be related to the study drugs.

The BeSt study, published in October 2005, was a randomized trial that examined 508 patients with recently diagnosed RA. Patients were divided into 4 groups. The first group received monotherapy, the second group received step-up combination therapy, the third group received combination therapy with tapered high-dose prednisone, and the fourth received initial combination therapy with infliximab. Nine patients in group 4 had latent TB and received isoniazid before infliximab. There were no new cases of TB or opportunistic infections reported in this study. Six patients in the infliximab group experienced SAEs, which included pulmonary embolism, septic arthritis, transient cardiac ischemia, peripheral vascular disease, MTX pneumonitis, and pneumonia.

Certolizumab is a recombinant polyethylene glycolylated fragment of a humanized anti-TNF monoclonal antibody with high affinity to TNF. The affinity of certolizumab for TNF-α is stronger than adalimumab and infliximab. The safety of certolizumab in RA has been evaluated in 7 major clinical trials. These clinical trials include FAST4-WARD,[25] RAPID 1,[26] RAPID 2,[27] Study 014,[28] REALISTIC,[29] CERTAIN,[30] and DOSE-FLEX.[31] In these studies treatment-emergent adverse events (AEs) occurred after the first time the subject received the study drug and for up to 12 weeks after the last dose.

The RAPID 1 trial was published in October 2008. This study investigated placebo versus treatment with 200 and 400 mg certolizumab pegol (CZP). The overall rate of treatment AEs for the placebo group was 125.9 per 100 patient-years. In the 200-mg CZP group it was 96.6 per 100 patient-years, and in the 400-mg CZP group it was 94.6 per patient-years. Most AEs were mild or moderate. Infections led to the withdrawal of the study drug in 6 patients in each of the CZP dosage groups. No patients in the placebo group discontinued the study drug due to infection. The most common infections reported were urinary tract infections, upper respiratory tract infections, and nasopharyngitis. Between the groups, the frequency of infectious AEs was comparable. SAEs were observed more frequently in the CZP groups than the placebo group. The most frequent serious infections were gastroenteritis, urinary tract infections, lower respiratory tract infections, and TB. SAEs occurred in 5.3 (per 100 patient-years) in the CZP 200 mg group, 7.3 in the 400 mg CZP group, and 2.2 in the placebo group. Five patients living in Eastern Europe who received CZP developed TB; 3 of whom had a positive PPD at baseline, another was a worker in a TB clinic. One hundred and seventy-two patients who had a PPD equal to or greater than 5 mm were enrolled in the study. Malignant neoplasms were found in 12 patients (1 receiving placebo [1.1 per 100 patient-years; thyroid neoplasm], 7 receiving 200 mg of CZP). There were no clinically or statistically significant differences between the 2 CZP dosage groups. The 8 instances of AEs related to death were deemed unrelated or unlikely to be related to CZP.

The FAST4WARD study was published in June 2009. There were no cases of opportunistic infections, including TB. No cases of systemic lupus erythematosus (SLE) were reported and there were no deaths.

The RAPID 2 trial was published in June 2009. The RAPID 2 trial again looked at CZP 200 and 400 mg and a placebo group. In the placebo group, 3.2% of patients experienced SAEs compared with 7.3% in the CZP group. Serious infections did not occur in the placebo group, whereas 3.2% of patients in the 200-mg CZP group and 2.4% of patients in the 400-mg CZP group were affected. Serious infections included erysipelas, TB, gastroenteritis, tooth abscess, postoperative wound infection, and urosepsis. Five patients in total developed TB and they were in the CZP group. One case of malignant neoplasm occurred in each group. Two patients died during the study, both from the CZP groups. Neither of the deaths were reported as related to the study drug.

Study 014 was published in July 2012. This study investigated patients receiving CZP with MTX and those receiving placebo with MTX. SAEs were reported in 12.9% of patients in the CZP + MTX group and 10.1% of patients in the placebo + MTX group. The rates of infections were higher in the CZP + MTZ group (26.6%), which was statistically significant ($P = .026$), in comparison with the MTX + placebo group (14.3%). Serious infections were reported in 3 patients in the CZP + MTX group and 2 patients in the MTX + placebo group. There were no cases of TB, malignancies, SLE, or deaths in the study.

The REALISTIC study was published in December 2012. They compared CZP versus placebo. The most common SAEs were infections in 2.6% of patients in the

CZP group and 1.9% of patients in the placebo group. There were 2 cases of *Aspergillus* infection in the CZP group. There were no cases of TB. There were 4 cases of malignant neoplasms in the CZP group. These neoplasms included carcinoid tumor, adenocarcinoma of the pancreas, skin melanoma, and uterine sarcoma. There were 2 malignant neoplasms in the placebo group: breast cancer and skin melanoma. There were 2 deaths in the CZP group. One death was because of sigmoid diverticulitis and the other because of necrotizing pneumonia, and both deaths were stated to possibly be related to CZP.

The CERTAIN trial, published in December 2013, investigated CZP and placebo groups. The rates of each type of AE were comparable in both groups. SAEs were reported in 5.2% of patients in the CZP group. These included irritable bowel syndrome, otitis media, polyarthritis, RA, sepsis, and disc protrusion. SAEs were reported in 7.1% of patients in the placebo group. These included pneumonia, tendon rupture, joint effusion, cerebrovascular accident, Wegener's, pleurisy, breast cancer, and basal cell carcinoma.

The DOSEFLEX trial was published in February 2015 and examined patients who received CZP. The most common AEs were infections, which were present in 54% of patients. The most common infections were upper respiratory tract infections. SAEs were found in 8.7% of patients. The most common SAE was infection, followed by connective tissue disorders and cardiac disorders. There was 1 case of malignant melanoma and 1 case of basal cell carcinoma. There were no deaths and no reported cases of TB.

In a Cochrane meta-analysis of 22 randomized controlled trials from 2002 to 2012, cetrolizumab was found to have a relative risk of 2.29, which was comparable with the relative risk of other TNF-α inhibitors. However, this study was limited because there were fewer patients treated with certolizumab compared with some of the other TNF-α inhibitors.[32] Also, when compared with the other TNF-α inhibitors in this study, CZP was not associated with an increased risk of malignancies, infections, or cardiovascular events.[33] The opportunistic infections that were studied in this review were TB, oral or esophageal candidiasis, herpes simplex, herpes zoster, Epstein-Barr virus, *Nocardia*, and cytomegalovirus.

Golimumab, or Simponi, is a human anti-TNF drug that was approved by the FDA in 2009 for the treatment of RA, ankylosing spondylitis, and psoriatic arthritis. There were 2 large, double-blinded, randomized trials that investigated the efficacy and safety of golimumab in patients with RA: the GO-BEFORE[34] and GO-FORWARD[35] studies.

The GO-BEFORE study was published in June 2008, and separated patients into 4 groups; group 1 patients received MTX plus placebo, group 2 received golimumab 100 mg plus placebo, group 3 received golimumab 50 mg plus MTX, group 4 received golimumab 100 mg plus MTX. The most common SAEs were pneumonia, anemia, and serious infections. SAEs were reported in 6.9%, 3.2%, 6.3%, and 6.3%, respectively, of the 4 groups. Tuberculosis of the spine was diagnosed in a patient in group 2, 33 days after she received golimumab. However, the spinal lesion was present before the patient started the study. Two patients died during the study; neither were attributed to the study drug. Malignancies developed in 4 patients; 1 with Hodgkin lymphoma, 2 with breast cancer, and 1 with squamous cell skin cancer. Overall the incidence of SAEs and serious infections was low. However, there was a higher incidence of patients who developed serious infections in the golimumab 100 mg with MTX group in comparison with the other groups.

The GO-FORWARD study was published in December 2008 and separated patients into 4 groups. The groups varied on the dosages of golimumab and whether or not MTX was used. Patients were followed for 2 years, and 22.6% of golimumab-treated patients developed SAEs. Serious infections were the most common SAEs. Two patients in the 100 mg golimumab plus placebo group developed active TB, and 4 patients in the same group died during the 2-year duration of the study. The causes of death were sepsis, hepatic failure, circulatory insufficiency, and complicated respiratory distress following acute pulmonary edema, which occurred after open cholecystectomy. Two placebo-treated patients and 14 golimumab-treated patients developed malignancy.

OTHER CLASSES OF BIOLOGICS

TCZ targets the IL-6 receptor, thus inhibiting the inflammatory cascade. It is 1 of the newer biologics studied for the treatment of adult patients with RA with a refractory response to DMARDs. Because of its newer status the risk of infections with treatment of TCZ is less well studied. The 2 long-term extension studies that investigated the efficacy and safety of TCZ were the SUMMACTA[36] and the BREVACTA[37] trials.

SUMMACTA, published in January 2014, demonstrated a similar safety profile between intravenous and subcutaneous administration of TCZ. The rate of serious infections was 3.6 per 100 patient-years in the TCZ group versus 1.5 per 100 patient-years in the MTX group. The most common serious infections included pneumonia, urinary tract infection, cellulitis, herpes zoster, gastroenteritis, diverticulitis, sepsis, and bacterial sepsis.

The BREVACTA trial, published November 2014, was a 24-week, double-blinded study in patients with active RA and inadequate response to DMARDs. Patients received TCZ 162 mg or placebo every other week, and 4.6% of patients in the treatment group and 3.7% of patients in the placebo group experienced SAEs. The most common SAE was infection in both groups. Three patients died during the study, all in the TCZ group, and the deaths were reported as related to the drug. Deaths were from *Haemophilus influenzae* sepsis, sepsis secondary to gastrointestinal causes, and complications of a lower respiratory tract infection, respectively. Three malignancies occurred in the treatment group, which were deemed unrelated to the study medication.

Rituximab is an anticluster of differentiation 20 (CD20) monoclonal antibody that recognizes B cell linage from the pro-B cell onward. Cell death is caused by complement-mediated and antibody-mediated cytotoxicity targeting peripheral B cells. It is used to treat patients with RA, but also leukemia, lymphoma, and antibody-driven disorders such as hemolytic anemia and systemic lupus erythematosus. Although there have been reported cases of patients on rituximab who developed serious infections, these individuals were also treated with biologic agents and/or TNF-α inhibitors.[3] An increased risk of infection is evident in patients with lymphoma or other hematological malignancies on rituximab maintenance therapy, but no similar data exist for patients with RA.[38] Progressive multifocal leukoencephalopathy is an opportunistic central nervous system (CNS) infection that may develop in 1 per 25,000 patients with RA treated with rituximab.[39]

Abatacept is a T cell co-stimulator modulator with CTLA-4 linked to human IgG1. It blocks binding of CD80/CD86 to T cell CD28 and therefore blocks co-stimulation.[40] The incidence of serious infections was roughly 2% over 26 weeks and 2.5% to 3% in more than 1 year of medication use.[40] In a trial that compared the use of abatacept with MTX and infliximab, versus MTX as a sole treatment, there was a lower rate of serious infections with abatacept treatment.[41] In a meta-analysis the incidence of serious infections in patients with RA taking abatacept was 2.5%, which was not a significant increase.

REACTIVATION OF LATENT TUBERCULOSIS AND OTHER INFECTIONS

The reactivation of latent TB is a well-studied infectious adverse effect of TNF-α inhibitors.[3] However, etanercept has lower risk of causing reactivation TB than either infliximab or adalimumab.[14] Individuals with TB on TNF inhibitors are more likely to develop extrapulmonary and CNS complications, such as meningitis and tuberculomas.[3] Also, after looking at long-term follow-up data on patients who developed TB after taking TNF-α inhibitors, it seems that biological therapy can be safely resumed after treatment of TB.[42,43] The risk for reactivation of latent TB with abatecept and TCZ seems to be low; however, there are fewer clinical trials that used these drugs and included a population with TB exposure or had TB screening as a part of their studies.[41]

The risk of patients developing reactivation TB can be mitigated by appropriate screening for, and treatment of, latent TB infection when starting patients on anti-TNF therapy.[3] Tuberculin skin test, interferon gamma release assay, chest radiograph, and sputum examination are all useful screening tools to supplement the exposure history and physical examination findings in decreasing the incidence of reactivation TB in immunocompromised patients on TNF-α inhibitors.

Biologic therapy is also believed to increase the risk of atypical mycobacterial infections, *Legionella*, *Listeria*, and *Salmonella*, as well as viral and fungal infections. Histoplasmosis is the most common fungal infection associated with TNF inhibitors.[3] CNS involvement and disseminated disease is more likely in patients with histoplasmosis on TNF-α inhibitors. However, in a retrospective study of 98 patients treated with TNF-α inhibitors who developed histoplasmosis, only 2% developed CNS involvement.[3] Other patients with possible endemic mycoses on TNF-α inhibitors are increasingly susceptible to coccidiomycois and blastomycosis. Herpesvirus and *Listeria* and *Nocardia* meningitis are rare but reported infections associated with TNF-α inhibitor use[3]

Children are especially vulnerable to bacterial infections because of the immaturity of their immune system. In a study examining children with JIA who used TNF-α inhibitors, the risk of serious bacterial infections requiring hospitalization was 2.7 times greater than children with JIA who were treated with DMARDs.[5] Although DMARDs and TNF-α inhibitors are often used together, the risk of infection is also associated with TNF-α inhibitors being used as a monotherapy in children with JIA.[5]

Although it is evident that biologics result in secondary immune deficiency, the significant benefits of these medications need to be considered as well. TNF-α inhibitors are used in the treatment of children with moderately to severely active polyarticular JIA, which causes arthritis involving more than 4 joints within the first 6 months in patients younger than 16 years. These patients generally have a refractory course and are therefore more likely to have joint damage, which negatively affects their functioning and quality of life. With the advent of biologic agents, the disease course and prognosis has dramatically changed for those affected.[44] TNF-α inhibitors have been shown to decrease disease remission. Starting TNF-α inhibitors earlier in the disease course of RA and JIA has been shown to improve outcome in clinical studies.[45,46]

There are measures that providers can take to reduce the risks of infection. Reducing the dose of glucocorticoids, alternate-day dosing, and concurrent use of other immunosuppressive medications can decrease associated risks.[47] The US FDA and the European Medicines Agency have developed parameters for administering biologics for adult patients.[5] However, there needs to be guidelines for the screening of children being treated with TNF-α inhibitors (**Table 1**).

Table 1
List of biologics and their infection risk

Biologic	Brand Name	Mechanism of Action	Approved Uses	Infection Risk
Certolizumab	Cimzia	TNF-α inhibitor; binds to human TNF-α with a K_D of 90 pM	Crohn disease, RA, psoriatic arthritis, ankylosing spondylitis, plaque psoriasis	Increased risk of opportunistic infections. Cases of reactive TB or new TB have occurred. Most common adverse reactions >7% (upper respiratory tract infection, rash, and urinary tract infection). New infection risk 0.91 per patient-year in RA patients.[48]
Adalimumab	Humira	TNF-α inhibitor; binds to human TNF-α	RA, psoriatic arthritis, ankylosing spondylitis, ulcerative colitis	Increased risk of serious infection. Cases of reactive TB or new TB have occurred.[49]
Infliximab	Remicade	TNF-α inhibitor; chimeric human and mouse peptide sequence monoclonal antibody	RA, Crohn disease, ankylosing spondylitis, psoriatic arthritis, plaque psoriasis, ulcerative colitis	Most common adverse reactions (>10%), infections. Treated serious infections reported in 36% patients. Most common, sinusitis, pharyngitis, bronchitis, and urinary tract infections. Serious infections included pneumonia, cellulitis, abscess, skin ulceration, sepsis, and bacterial infection. Cases of reactivation of TB or new TB infections have been observed.[50]
Golimumab	Simponi	TNF-α inhibitor	RA, psoriatic arthritis, ankylosing spondylitis, ulcerative colitis	Serious infections have been reported in 1.4% of treated patients. Serious infections include sepsis, pneumonia, cellulitis, abscess, TB, invasive fungal infections, and hepatitis B infection. Cases of reactivation of TB or new TB infections have been observed.[51]
Rituximab	Rituxan	B cell inhibitor	RA, Wegener's granulomatosis, pemphigus vulgaris, non-Hodgkin lymphoma, chronic lymphocytic leukemia	Serious infections have been reported in patients with prolonged hypogammaglobulinemia. Most common infections, nasopharyngitis, upper respiratory tract infections, urinary tract infections, bronchitis, and sinusitis.[52]

(continued on next page)

Table 1
(continued)

Biologic	Brand Name	Mechanism of Action	Approved Uses	Infection Risk
Anakinra	Kineret	IL-1 Inhibitor	RA	Incidence of infection was 40% in Kineret-treated patients, vs 35% in placebo-treated patients. Incidence of serious infections, 1.8% in Kineret-treated patients vs 0.6% in placebo. Most common infections, cellulitis, pneumonia, and bone and joint infections. Patients with asthma were at higher risk of developing infection (5%) vs placebo (<1%).[53]
Sarilumab	Kevzara	IL-6 inhibitor	RA	Serious infections have been reported. Most frequent pneumonia and cellulitis. Rate of overall infection 0.6%–0.8% in the treatment group compared with 0.5% in the placebo group. Rate of serious infection in events per 100 patient-years was 3.0 (150 mg) and 4.3 (200 mg) in the Kevzara treatment groups compared with 3.1 in the placebo group. Cases of TB have been reported.[54]
Tocilizumab	Actemra	IL-6 Inhibitor	RA, giant cell arteritis, polyarticular JIA, systemic JIA, cytokine release syndrome	Rate of overall infections, 119 events per 100 patient-years, similar to the MTX group. Serious infections, 3.6 per 100 patient-years, 1.5 per patient-years in the MTX group. Most common infections, upper respiratory tract infections and nasopharyngitis. Most common serious infections, pneumonia, urinary tract infection (UTI), cellulitis, herpes zoster. Cases of TB have been reported.[55]
Abatacept	Orencia	CTLA4 co-stimulator inhibitor	RA	Infections reported in 54% patients in the treatment group, 48% in the placebo group. Most common infections, upper respiratory tract infections, nasopharyngitis, sinusitis, UTI, influenza, bronchitis. Serious infections, 3% in the treatment group, 1.9% patients in the placebo group.[40]

Note: Approved uses are in the United States indicated by the FDA.

REFERENCES

1. Keyser FD. Choice of biologic therapy for patients with rheumatoid arthritis: the infection perspective. Curr Rheumatol Rev 2011;7(1):77–87.
2. Rutherford AI, Patarata E, Subesinghe S, et al. Opportunistic infections in rheumatoid arthritis patients exposed to biologic therapy: results from the British Society for Rheumatology Biologics Register for Rheumatoid Arthritis. Rheumatology 2018;57(6):997–1001.
3. Bradshaw MJ, Cho TA, Chow FC. Central nervous system infections associated with immunosuppressive therapy for rheumatic disease. Rheum Dis Clin North Am 2017;43(4):607–19.
4. Carneiro C, Bloom R, Ibler E, et al. Rate of serious infection in patients who are prescribed systemic biologic or nonbiologic agents for psoriasis: a large, single center, retrospective, observational cohort study. Dermatol Ther 2017;30(5). https://doi.org/10.1111/dth.12529.
5. Lee WJ, Lee TA, Suda KJ, et al. Risk of serious bacterial infection associated with tumour necrosis factor-alpha inhibitors in children with juvenile idiopathic arthritis. Rheumatology 2018;57(2):273–82.
6. Zhang JM, An J. Cytokines, inflammation, and pain. Int Anesthesiol Clin 2007; 45(2):27–37.
7. Leonardi CL, Powers JL, Matheson RT, et al. Etanercept as monotherapy in patients with psoriasis. N Engl J Med 2003;349:2014–22.
8. Papp KA. Etanercept in psoriasis. Expert Opin Pharmacother 2004;5:2139–46.
9. Keystone EC. Safety of biologic therapies—an update. J Rheumatol Suppl 2005; 74:8–12.
10. Kavanaugh A, Tutuncu Z, Catalan-Sanchez T. Update on anti-tumor necrosis factor therapy in the spondyloarthropathies including psoriatic arthritis. Curr Opin Rheumatol 2006;18:347–53.
11. Klareskog L, van der Heijde D, de Jager JP, et al. TEMPO (Trial of Etanercept and Methotrexate with Radiographic Patient Outcomes) study investigators Therapeutic effect of the combination of etanercept and methotrexate compared with each treatment alone in patients with rheumatoid arthritis: double-blind randomised controlled trial. Lancet 2004;363(9410):675–81.
12. Emery P, et al. Comparison of methotrexate monotherapy with a combination of methotrexate and etanercept in active, early, moderate to severe rheumatoid arthritis (COMET): a randomised, double-blind, parallel treatment trial. Lancet 2008;372(9636):375–82.
13. Rutherford AI, Subesinghe S, Hyrich KL, et al. Serious infection across biologic-treated patients with rheumatoid arthritis: results from the British Society for Rheumatology Biologics Register for Rheumatoid Arthritis. Ann Rheum Dis 2018;77: 905–10.
14. Tubach F, Salmon D, Ravaud P, et al. Risk of tuberculosis is higher with anti-tumor necrosis factor monoclonal antibody therapy than with soluble tumor necrosis factor receptor therapy: the three-year prospective French Research Axed on Tolerance of Biotherapies registry. Arthritis Rheum 2009;60(7):1884–94.
15. Moreland LW, Weinblatt ME, Keystone EC, et al. Etanercept treatment in adults with established rheumatoid arthritis: 7 years of clinical experience. J Rheumatol 2006;33(5):854–61.
16. Sokka T. Rheumatoid arthritis databases. Rheum Dis Clin North Am 2004;30: 769–81, vi.

17. Salfeld J, Kaymakçalan Z, Tracey D, et al. Generation of fully human anti-TNF antibody D2E7 [abstract]. Arthritis Rheum 1998;41(Suppl 9):S57.

18. Weinblatt ME, Keystone EC, Furst DE, et al. Adalimumab, a fully human anti-tumor necrosis factor a monoclonal antibody for the treatment of RA in patients taking concomitant methotrexate. The ARMADA trial. Arthritis Rheum 2003;48: 35–45.

19. Keystone EC, Kavanaugh AF, Sharp JT, et al. Radiographic, clinical, and functional outcomes of treatment with adalimumab (a human anti-tumor necrosis factor monoclonal antibody) in patients with active rheumatoid arthritis receiving concomitant methotrexate therapy: a randomized, placebo-controlled, 52-week trial. Arthritis Rheum 2004;50(5):1400–11.

20. Van de Putte LB, Atkins C, Malaise M, et al. Efficacy and safety of adalimumab as monotherapy in patients with rheumatoid arthritis for whom previous disease modifying antirheumatic drug treatment has failed. Ann Rheum Dis 2004;63: 508–16.

21. Furst DE, Schiff MH, Fleischmann RM, et al. Efficacy and safety of the fully human anti-tumour necrosis factor-monoclonal antibody, and concomitant standard antirheumatic therapy for the treatment of rheumatoid arthritis: results of STAR (Safety Trial of Adalimumab in Rheumatoid Arthritis). J Rheumatol 2003;30:2563–71.

22. St Clair EW, van de Heijde D, Smolen JS, et al, Active-Controlled Study of Patients Receiving Infliximab for the Treatment of Rheumatoid Arthritis of Early Onset Study Group. Combination of infliximab and methotrexate therapy for early rheumatoid arthritis. Arthritis Rheum 2004;50:3432–43.

23. Goekoop-Ruiterman YPM, de Vries-Bouwstra JK, Allaart CF, et al. Clinical and radiographic outcomes of four diferent treatment strategies in patients with early rheumatoid arthritis (the BeST study). Arthritis Rheum 2005;52:3381–90.

24. Lipsky PE, van der Heijde DMFM, St Clair EW, et al, Anti-Tumor Necrosis Factor Trial in Rheumatoid Arthritis with Concomitant Therapy Study Group. Infliximab and methotrexate in the treatment of rheumatoid arthritis. N Engl J Med 2000; 343:1594–602.

25. Fleischmann R, Vencovsky J, van Vollenhoven RF, et al. Efficacy and safety of certolizumab pegol monotherapy every 4 weeks in patients with rheumatoid arthritis failing previous disease-modifying antirheumatic therapy: the FAST4WARD study. Ann Rheum Dis 2008;68(6):805–11.

26. Keystone E, Heijde DV, Mason D Jr, et al. Certolizumab pegol plus methotrexate is significantly more effective than placebo plus methotrexate in active rheumatoid arthritis: findings of a fifty-two-week, phase III, multicenter, randomized, double-blind, placebo-controlled, parallel-group study (RAPID 1). Arthritis Rheum 2009;60(5):1249.

27. Smolen J, Landewé RB, Mease P, et al. Efficacy and safety of certolizumab pegol plus methotrexate in active rheumatoid arthritis: the RAPID 2 study. A randomised controlled trial. Ann Rheum Dis 2008;68(6):797–804.

28. Choy E, McKenna F, Vencovsky J, et al. Certolizumab pegol plus MTX administered every 4 weeks is effective in patients with RA who are partial responders to MTX. Rheumatology 2012;51(7):1226–34.

29. Weinblatt ME, Fleischmann R, Huizinga TWJ, et al. Efficacy and safety of certolizumab pegol in a broad population of patients with active rheumatoid arthritis: results from the REALISTIC phase IIIb study. Rheumatology 2012;51(12): 2204–14.

30. Smolen JS, Emery P, Ferraccioli GF, et al. Certolizumab pegol in rheumatoid arthritis patients with low to moderate activity: the CERTAIN double-blind, randomised, placebo-controlled trial. Ann Rheum Dis 2015;74:843–50.

31. Furst DE, Shaikh SA, Greenwald M, et al. Two dosing regimens of certolizumab pegol in patients with active rheumatoid arthritis. Arthritis Care Res (Hoboken) 2015;67(2):151–60.

32. Ford AC, Peyrin-Biroulet L. Opportunistic infections with anti-tumor necrosis factor-alpha therapy in inflammatory bowel disease: meta-analysis of randomized controlled trials. Am J Gastroenterol 2013;108:1268–76.

33. Harrold LR, Litman HJ, Saunders KC, et al. One-year risk of serious infection in patients treated with certolizumab pegol as compared with other TNF inhibitors in a real-world setting: Data from a national U.S. Rheumatoid arthritis registry. Arthritis Res Ther 2018;20:2.

34. Emery P, Fleischmann RM, Moreland LW, et al. Golimumab (GLM), a new human anti-TNF-α monoclonal antibody, administered subcutaneously (SC) every 4 weeks in methotrexate-naive patients with active rheumatoid arthritis (RA): a randomized, double-blind, placebo-controlled, GO-BEFORE study [abstract no. THU0138]. 2008 Annual European Congress of rheumatology; Paris, Jun 11–14, 2008.

35. Keystone EC, Genovese MC, Klareskog L, et al. Golimumab, a human antibody to TNF-α given by monthly subcutaneous injections, in active rheumatoid arthritis despite methotrexate: the GO-FORWARD study. Ann Rheum Dis 2009;68(6): 789–96.

36. Burmester GR, Rubbert-Roth A, Cantagrel A, et al. A randomised, double-blind, parallel-group study of the safety and efficacy of subcutaneous tocilizumab versus intravenous tocilizumab in combination with traditional disease-modifying antirheumatic drugs in patients with moderate to severe rheumatoid arthritis (SUMMACTA study). Ann Rheum Dis 2013;73(1):69–74.

37. Kivitz A, Olech E, Borofsky M, et al. Subcutaneous tocilizumab versus placebo in combination with disease-modifying antirheumatic drugs in patients with rheumatoid arthritis. Arthritis Care Res (Hoboken) 2014;66(11):1653–61.

38. Al-Tawfiq JA, Al-Khatti AA. Disseminated systemic Nocardia farcinica infection complicating alefacept and infliximab therapy in a patient with severe psoriasis. Int J Infect Dis 2010;14(2):e153–7.

39. Clifford DB, Ances B, Costello C, et al. Rituximab-associated progressive multifocal leukoencephalopathy in rheumatic arthritis. Arch Neurol 2011;68(9): 1156–64.

40. Orencia [FDA label]. Princeton (NJ): Bristol-Myers Squibb Company; 2005. Available at: https://www.accessdata.fda.gov/drugsatfda_docs/label/2005/125118lbl.pdf.

41. Kremer JM, Genant HK, Moreland LW, et al. Effects of abatacept in patients with methotrexate-resistant active rheumatoid arthritis: a randomized trial. Ann Intern Med 2006;144:865–76.

42. Denis B, Lefort A, Flipo RM, et al. Long-term follow-up of patients with tuberculosis as a complication of tumour necrosis factor (TNF)-alpha antagonist therapy: safe re-initiation of TNF-alpha blockers after appropriate anti-tuberculous treatment. Clin Microbiol Infect 2008;14:183–6.

43. Kremer JM, Genant HK, Moreland LW, et al. Results of a two-year follow up study of patients with rheumatoid arthritis who received a combination of abatacept and methotrexate. Arthritis Rheum 2008;58:953–63.

44. Oberle EJ, Harris JG, Verbsky JW. Polyarticular juvenile idiopathic arthritis – epidemiology and management approaches. Clin Epidemiol 2014;6:379–93.

45. Giannini E, Ruperto N, Ravelli A, et al. Preliminary definition of improvement in juvenile arthritis. Arthritis Rheum 1997;40(7):1202–9.

46. Tynjala P, Vahasalo P, Tarkiainen M, et al. Aggressive combination drug therapy in very early polyarticular juvenile idiopathic arthritis (ACUTE-JIA): a multicenter randomized open-label clinical trial. Ann Rheum Dis 2011;70(9):1605–12.

47. Fauci AS. Alternate-day corticosteroid therapy. Am J Med 1978;64(5):729–31.

48. Cimzia [FDA label]. Smyrna (GA): UCB, Inc; 2016. Available at: https://www.accessdata.fda.gov/drugsatfda_docs/label/2017/125160s270lbl.pdf.

49. Abbott Laboratories. Humira [FDA label]. North Chicago (IL): Abbott Laboratories; 2008. Available at: https://www.accessdata.fda.gov/drugsatfda_docs/label/2008/125057s0110lbl.pdf.

50. Janssen Biotech, Inc. Remicaid [FDA label]. Horsham (PA): Janssen Biotech, Inc; 2013. Available at: https://www.accessdata.fda.gov/drugsatfda_docs/label/2013/103772s5359lbl.pdf.

51. Janssen Biotech, Inc. Simponi [FDA label]. Horsham (PA): Janssen Biotech, Inc; 2011. Available at: https://www.accessdata.fda.gov/drugsatfda_docs/label/2011/125289s0064lbl.pdf.

52. Genentech, Inc. Rituxan [FDA label]. San Francisco (CA): Genentech, Inc; 2010. Available at: https://www.accessdata.fda.gov/drugsatfda_docs/label/2010/103705s5311lbl.pdf.

53. Kineret [FDA label]. Stolkholm (Sweden): Swedish Orphan Biovitrum AB; 2015. Available at: https://www.accessdata.fda.gov/drugsatfda_docs/label/2016/103950s5175lbl.pdf.

54. Kevzara [FDA label]. Bridewater (NJ): Sanofi-Aventis; 2017. Available at: https://www.accessdata.fda.gov/drugsatfda_docs/label/2017/761037s000lbl.pdf.

55. Actemra [FDA label]. San Francisco (CA): Genentech, Inc; 2017. Available at: https://www.accessdata.fda.gov/drugsatfda_docs/label/2010/125276lbl.pdf.

New Insights and Treatments in Atopic Dermatitis

Shweta Saini, MD, Milind Pansare, MD*

KEYWORDS

- Atopic dermatitis • Topical and systemic treatments • Small molecule inhibitors
- Biologics • Atopic dermatitis phenotypes

KEY POINTS

- Atopic dermatitis (AD) is complex chronic inflammatory skin disorder.
- There is now an increased understanding of the pathogenesis of AD, resulting in discovery of much wanted new targeted therapies.
- Various AD phenotypes and endotypes are described, enabling targeted therapies in the future.
- Whether a long-term cure or sustained benefits will occur remains to be seen.

INTRODUCTION

Atopic dermatitis (AD) is the most common inflammatory skin disease, with significant morbidity. The disease affects 20% to 30% of children and 7% to 10% of adults.[1] It is characterized by chronic itching, dry skin, eczematous lesions, and relapsing course. Pruritus is the sine quo non feature, causing a significant disruption of daily life. In many patients with moderate to severe AD, a chronic itch-scratch cycle causes significant morbidities such as sleep loss, impaired quality of life, and psychosocial problems, besides complications including skin infections.[2] The frequent need for treatment creates significant financial and mental burdens on families.[3] AD is also the first evidence of atopic disease in early childhood, with likely development of the atopic march of allergic rhinitis, asthma, and food allergies in these patients causing further morbidities.[2] Recent studies also link AD to other nonallergic conditions, including a risk for systemic and multiorgan infections,[4] cardiovascular diseases (coronary artery disease),[5] and neuropsychiatric disorders such as depression, anxiety, and attention-deficit/hyperactivity disorders.[5]

The treatment of AD has evolved slowly from using topical emollients in the early 1930s to topical steroids (1960s) and calcineurin inhibitors (2000s), and now, after a

[a] Division of Allergy and Immunology, Department of Pediatrics, Wayne State University, Children's Hospital of Michigan, Pediatric Specialty Center, Suite # 4018, 3950 Beaubien Boulevard, Detroit, MI 48201, USA
* Corresponding author.
E-mail address: mpansare@dmc.org

Pediatr Clin N Am 66 (2019) 1021–1033
https://doi.org/10.1016/j.pcl.2019.06.008
0031-3955/19/© 2019 Elsevier Inc. All rights reserved.

long wait, new biologic agents are available (2016), such as anti–interleukin (IL) 4/IL-13 antibodies. Some of the newer therapies are discussed in this article.

PATHOPHYSIOLOGY

AD is a complex skin inflammatory disorder with multifactorial cause, including a complex interaction of epidermal barrier defects, immune dysregulation of both adaptive and innate immunity, and environmental.[6,7] There is ongoing debate triggers whether AD is a consequence of genetic mutations affecting the epidermal barrier (outside-in model) or is caused by inflammation inhibiting epidermal differentiation (inside-out model).[6] Importantly, immune activation is not only seen in AD skin but also in clinically normal-appearing skin, as well with AD-specific inflammatory changes in blood components suggesting the systemic aspect of this disease.[7,8] AD is understood to be primarily a T cell–driven disease; with a dominant T helper (TH) type 2 immune response with increased levels of IL-4, IL-13, IL-31, and chemokine ligand 18 (CCL18) cytokines and additional activation of TH22, TH17/IL-23, and TH1 cytokine pathways.[8] The lesional levels of these cytokines were shown to be significantly increased compared with healthy skin.[7,8] The IL-4 and IL-13 cytokines are produced by TH2 cells and play a key role in the pathogenesis of AD and also overproduction of immunoglobulin (Ig) E.[8–10] Filagrin (FLG), loricrin, and involucrin are downregulated in both lesional and nonlesional skin by IL-4 and IL-13, contributing to a defective skin barrier and thereby penetration of allergens and bacteria, leading to allergen sensitization and infections, which is a hallmark of AD.[7,9] IL-4 and IL-13 also inhibit production of antimicrobial peptides predisposing to *Staphylococcus aureus* infections, further enhancing skin inflammation and barrier defects.[10,11] The IL-4/IL-13–driven inflammation can also downregulate the TH1 (interferon gamma) and TH-17 (IL-17)–dependent skin defense mechanism.[8,12] Although IL-17 is increased AD lesions, its antimicrobial effects are inhibited in the presence of IL-4/IL-13.[12] TH-17 also contributes to immune dysregulation as well as barrier abnormalities by downregulating FLG cellular adhesion molecules.[12] In chronic AD, TH2 and TH22 responses are also increased with parallel activation of the TH1 axis.[8] IL-22 is identified as the key mediator for epidermal hyperplasia, whereas the IL-31 cytokine is associated with itch and correlates with disease severity.[8] The chronic inflammation in the skin with various triggers and accentuated by defects in the skin barrier results in relapsing clinical rash and itching.

CLINICAL FEATURES

Different phenotypes of AD are now described based on IgE levels (intrinsic and extrinsic), age (pediatric and adult AD), FLG gene mutation, race, or ethnicity (Asian and European/American). Extrinsic AD is characterized by increase in total IgE (both total and allergen specific), high eosinophil count, and family history of atopic disease, whereas intrinsic AD shows normal IgE levels and lack of atopic history in the patient or in the patient's family.[13] Both show strong TH2 activation; however, in intrinsic AD there is stronger activation of TH17 and TH22 axis.[13] Pediatric AD has early onset, extensor surface involvement, a different skin microbiome,[14] and much higher levels of activated cytokines in nonlesional skin in children.[15] Ethnic differences are also seen, with Asian AD showing more parakeratosis, significantly increased TH17 axis, and cytokine profile suggesting a blend of AD and psoriasis.[16] In adult AD, FLG deficiency is common and also the peripheral blood shows TH22 polarization, unlike in child AD with TH2 dominance.[14] FLG gene mutation has been associated with a more severe and persistent form of AD but is seen in only 30% of European patients and is rare in African Americans.[17] Patients with FLG gene mutation have also been shown to outgrow their disease with age, suggesting the complexity of AD.[17] Recognizing different endotypes/phenotypes of AD will be important to customize therapies as new targeted agents are discovered in the future.

MANAGEMENT

The goal of treatment in AD is to reduce symptoms, prevent exacerbations, treat superinfection, minimize treatment risks, and restore the integrity of the skin. In most patients with mild disease, treatment goals are achieved with topical therapies alone, unlike in patients with moderate to severe disease, whose management is challenging.

The general principles of therapy include education and active participation of patients and their families, improving hydration and skin barrier function, eliminating exacerbating factors, and treatment of skin inflammation. At present a guideline-based or stepped-care approach for treating AD is lacking. Thus, in clinical practice, there are distinct approaches to management, and varied advice and recommendations are given to patients by both primary care providers and specialists. This

Table 1 Management of Atopic dermatitis-Basic and Step-up treatments	
Basic Management	**Step-up Treatment**
1. Skin hydration	1. Mild-moderate AD
a. Bathing: warm baths or showers with nonsoap cleansers	Basic management plus:
b. Moisturizers: prompt, frequent, and liberal use of preservative-free and fragrance-free moisturizers	a. Topical antiinflammatory therapies
2. Allergen avoidance	a. Acute and/or maintenance treatments
a. Food is not common, as often considered	i. Topical corticosteroids
b. Need to confirm with oral challenge	- Active: acute flare
c. Extensive testing and food elimination not recommended	Appropriate potency for 3–4 weeks with stepdown to lower potency for additional few weeks until improved
d. Additives rare cause	Proactive: in AD flare areas
e. Environment: dust mites, aeroallergen	2–3 times a week for months
3. Elimination of triggers	ii. Topical calcineurin inhibitors
a. Known irritants	Recommended for >2 y of age, steroid sparing
b. harsh fabrics-wool	Useful for Facial AD
c. Irritants: soap/cleansers, fragrance	iii. Newer agents: crisaborole
d. Extreme temperatures	b. Adjuvants
e. Pollutants	a. Antihistamines: oral
4. WWT and alternative clothing	b. Weigh pros/cons of use
a. WWT acutely and for maintenance	c. Infections: bacterial, viral, fungal
b. Derma Silk, silk Skinnies	a. Antiseptic measures: dilute bleach baths
	b. Specific infections: antibiotics or antivirals
	2. Moderate-severe AD
	All of the above plus:
	1. Newer agents: biologics
	2. Systemic immunomodulating agents
	3. Phototherapy
	4. Allergen immunotherapy
	5. Anti-IgE therapy
	6. Hospitalization

Abbreviation: WWT, wet wrap therapy.

variation causes confusion and angst for patient and families while dealing with a chronic and frustrating condition.

Good clinical management should include 2 elements: (1) basic management, and (2) step-up treatment of severe AD. Some salient features are listed in **Table 1** and **Box 1**. This article focuses on newer therapeutics, but the importance of good basic management cannot be overlooked for successful outcomes for treatment of AD. Readers are recommended to read guidance documents about patient evaluation, treatment algorithms published by the American Academy of Dermatology as well as the American Academy of Allergy, Asthma, and Immunology.[18–21]

Box 1
Bathing instructions for patients with atopic dermatitis[19]

1. Bathing is suggested for both treatment and maintenance

2. No standard for frequency and duration is established

3. Regular once-daily bathing with warm (not hot) water of short duration (5–10 minutes)

4. Limited use of nonsoap cleansers that are neural to low pH, hypoallergenic, and fragrance free

5. Generous and frequent application of moisturizers, with first soon after bathing, to improve skin hydration

6. Soak and seal: soak skin in warm water for 15 minutes, light pat dry, and seal in moisturizer for severe AD

Step-up Treatments

Severe AD is a frustrating disease with a chronic and relapsing course with complications. Step-up therapies should only be considered in patients who are adherent and unimproved with vigorous, topical antiinflammatory therapies without underlying infections and in whom an alternate diagnosis is excluded. Until recently the treatment options were limited to phototherapy, systemic immunomodulatory agents, or immunotherapy, which are not evidence based and are limited because of side effects. The US Food and Drug Administration (FDA) recently approved a new biologic agent for treatment of chronic AD in adults. Many new targeted therapeutics, including small molecule agents and anticytokine proteins, are being investigated for treatment of AD, as listed in **Table 2**.

Small molecule agents

Crisaborole is low-molecular-weight boron-based compound (benzoxaborole) with effective penetration in human skin. It is a phosphodiesterase 4 (PDE4) inhibitor with topical antiinflammatory activity in skin. PDE4 activity is increased in AD skin, resulting in decreased intracellular levels of cyclic adenosine monophosphate, which results in increased production of proinflammatory cytokines.[22] Crisaborole has been shown to decrease PDE4 levels and inflammation in animal models. It is rapidly and substantially metabolized to inactive molecules, thus limiting the systemic effects. The clinical efficacy and safety of crisaborole 2% ointment were established in 2 large, randomized controlled, phase 3 clinical trials in the United States involving a total of 1522 subjects ($\geq$2 years old) with mild (Investigator's Static Global Assessment score [ISGA] score 2) to moderate (ISGA score 3) AD at baseline. Most subjects (87%) were children and adolescents (2–17 years old), with approximately (33%) 2 to 6 years old. The primary efficacy variable was an ISGA score of clear or almost clear skin or an

Table 2
New investigational agents for treatment of moderate to severe atopic dermatitis[25]

Target	Compound	Trial Phase, Clinicaltrials.gov Identifier
Topical Agents		
AhR	Tapinarof/Benvitimod	2a, NCT02466152/NCT02564055
PDE4	Roflumilast	2a
JAK1, JAK3	Tofacitinib	2a, stopped
JAK1, JAK3	LEO 124249/JTE-052	2a
S aureus	Roseomonas mucosa bacteria	1/2 antecubital AD
S aureus	Coagulase-negative Staphylococcus	1/2 ventral arm AD
PDE4	Crisaborole	Clinical use
Biologics		
IL-4	Pitrakinra	2a
IL-5	Mepolizumab	2a
IL-12/23P40	Ustekinumab	2a, NCT01806662
IL-13	Tralokinumab	2 completed, NCT02347176
IL-13	Lebrikizumab	2 completed, NCT02340234
IL-4/1L-13R	Dupilumab	Approved for clinical use 2017
IL-17	Secukinumab	2, NCT02594098
IL-22	Fezakinumab (IV)	2, NCT01941537
IL-31R	Nemolizumab	2 complete, NCT01986933
IL-31	BMS-981164	1, NCT01614756
TSLP	Tezepelumab	1 complete, NCT00757042
TSLP-R	MK-8226	1, NCT01732510
IgE	QGE031/ligelizumab	2 complete, NCT01552629

Abbreviations: AhR, aryl hydrocarbon receptor; IV, intravenous; JAK, Janus kinase; PDE, phosphodiesterase; TSLP, thymic stromal lymphopoietin; TSLP-R, thymic stromal lymphopoietin receptor.

improvement grade of at least 2 from baseline at the end of the 28-day period of twice-daily application of crisaborole.[23] In the 2 trials, crisaborole 2% ointment ameliorated disease severity as soon as day 8 of treatment, and produced rapid and sustained lessening of pruritus, which is an important morbidity for patients with AD. These outcomes were significant despite a strong vehicle effect relating to the benefits of emollient treatment and placebo response rates. A side effect directly implicated was application site pain (burning, stinging), occurred in at least 1% of patients.[23,24]

Crisaborole 2%, a topical nonsteroidal ointment, was approved by the FDA in 2016 for treatment of mild to moderate AD in patients aged at least 2 years. The improved risk-benefit profile makes it suitable for steroid-phobic patients and as a steroid-sparing agent. It can be used as first line of treatment or for long durations of maintenance therapy in place of topical steroids, and thus avoiding steroid side effects.

Biologic agents
Various anticytokine agents are being aggressively investigated for treatment of AD.[25] One agent was recently approved for clinical use.

Interleukin-4/interleukin-13 blockade Dupilumab is a fully human monoclonal antibody (mAb) targeting the common alpha chain of IL-4 and IL-13 receptor, thus blocking signaling through these cytokines. In a landmark study of phase 1, 2, and 3 trials, dupilumab treatment was shown to decrease skin inflammation and improved epidermal-associated measures with a significant clinical improvement of AD as well as associated symptoms including pruritus, anxiety, and depression.[25,26] A 52-week efficacy and safety study of dupilumab added to a medium dose of topical steroids in adults also showed similar clinical benefits compared with placebo, as observed during the earlier trial of 16 weeks.[26–28] Headache, nasopharyngitis, injection site reactions, and conjunctivitis in particular were frequently reported symptoms during the trials. Hypersensitivity reactions, including urticaria and serum sickness–like reactions, were reported in 15 subjects in the trials.[27] At present, dupilumab is the only biologic drug approved by the FDA for systemic treatment of AD. It will be interesting to know its treatment effects for allergic asthma, allergic rhinitis, or eosinophil esophagitis caused by its effects on TH2 cytokines. The phase 3 Liberty Asthma Quest trial, a large controlled study, is evaluating dupilumab efficacy and safety in adult patients with uncontrolled, moderate to severe asthma with pending results.[29] These study results will enhance the rationale of using biologics for treatment of AD and coexisting allergic disease such as asthma.

Dupilumab received FDA approval in March 2017 for adult patients (>18 years old) with moderate to severe AD whose disease is not adequately controlled with topical prescription therapies or when those therapies are not advisable. It can be used with or without topical corticosteroids. Dupilumab is available as 300-mg/2-mL pre-filled injection to be self-administered as a subcutaneous injection. Initial dose is 600 mg subcutaneously followed by 300 mg given subcutaneously every 2 weeks. Injections can be self-administered at home, patients need not have autoinjectable epinephrine, and routine blood tests and laboratory monitoring are not currently required.[30] Current limitations for clinical use of dupilumab include age cutoff, cost, and insurance coverage. It is likely to be a safe and effective alternative to phototherapy or systemic immunosuppressant drugs in adults with unimproved moderate to severe AD with topical therapies. The postmarketing experience will help educate clinicians about its long-term safety, efficacy, and also dosing recommendations, and duration of treatment.

Other T-helper 2 cytokine blockade studies

Interleukin-13 blockade IL-13 is a key cytokine involved in the pathophysiology of several atopic diseases.[8] IL-13–mediated signaling is initiated by binding to IL-13Ra1, which then recruits IL-4Ra to form a heterodimeric receptor complex. IL-13 also binds to IL-13Ra2, thought to function as a decoy receptor. IL-13–neutralizing antibodies interfere with IL-13 binding to IL-13Ra1, IL-4Ra, and/or IL-13Ra2. Tralokinumab is a human recombinant IgG4 mAb that binds to IL-13 and blocks interaction with IL-13 receptors. Phase II trials with the anti–IL-13 antibodies tralokinumab and lebrikizumab have shown some clinical efficacy compared with placebo. A phase 2b, randomized, double-blinded, placebo-controlled, dose-ranging study to evaluate the efficacy and safety of 3 doses of tralokinumab administered by subcutaneous injection in adults with moderate to severe AD every 2 weeks for 12 weeks was completed, with pending results (NCT02347176, clinicaltrials.gov).[31,32]

Interleukin-5 blockade Blood eosinophil levels have been shown to increase in AD. IL-5 is a Th2 cytokine that is important for eosinophil recruitment. An mAb to human IL-5, mepolizumab, failed to show efficacy in patients with moderate to severe AD. In a randomized, placebo-controlled, parallel-group study of 18 patients treated with 2 single doses of mepolizumab (750 mg given 1 week apart) versus 22 patients treated with placebo, peripheral blood eosinophil levels were significantly reduced in the treatment group compared with placebo ($P<.05$). Clinical success was not achieved, as assessed by Physician's Global Assessment, SCORAD, pruritus scoring, or thymus and activation-regulated chemokine values in the mepolizumab-treated group compared with placebo.[33]

Interleukin-31 blockade IL-31 is a key pruritus-inducing cytokine that is upregulated in AD. The source of IL-31 in AD lesions has been debated; IL-31–positive cells were observed either as mononuclear infiltrating cells or as cluster of differentiation 11b (CD11b)–coexpressing cells with IL-31 receptor A detected in keratinocytes and nerve fibers in the dermis of AD and in the neurons of normal dorsal root ganglia.[34] Nemolizumab (CIM331) is a humanized anti–IL-31 receptor A mAb, binds to IL-31 receptor A, and inhibits IL-31 signaling.[35] It was shown to decrease pruritus and dermatitis, and to improve sleep and clinical scores in adult patients with moderate to severe AD compared with placebo in 12-week, phase II trial (part A, NCT01986933, clinicaltrials.gov). A 52-week, double-blind extension study (part B) to assess the long-term efficacy and safety of nemolizumab when injected subcutaneously every 4 weeks or every 8 weeks was completed recently. Nemolizumab when used for up to 64 weeks was shown to be efficacious and overall well tolerated in patients with moderate to severe AD.[36] Pruritus is the most frustrating symptom of AD, causing morbidities and also being difficult to control. It is hoped that this new therapy will improve this morbidity.

Other cytokines: T-helper 17, T-helper 22 pathways, interleukin-12, and interleukinIL-23 AD is primarily a TH2 activation disease but activation of other T-helper cells is variably detected in other AD populations.TH1 pathway activation is increased in some adults with chronic AD, and low activation levels are also reported in acute lesions and in some early-onset AD in children. Some Asian AD populations showed additional Th17 activation as well as in some early-onset pediatric AD.[16] Th22 is another pathway upregulated in AD. IL22 was shown to inhibit epidermal differentiation and thus promote barrier defects. The significance of these pathways will perhaps be revealed by studies of Th17 blockade (NCT02594098, clinicaltrials.gov) and the anti–IL-22 antibody fezakinumab (NCT01941537, clinicaltrials.gov) currently in phase 2 clinical trials.[37]

Ustekinumab, a fully human mAb approved for the treatment of psoriasis and psoriatic arthritis, binds to the common p40 subunit of IL-12/IL-23. These cytokines are produced by inflammatory myeloid cells and play a key role in the development of TH1 and TH17 cells.[37] In patients with AD, Weiss and colleagues[38] found that treatment with ustekinumab resulted in a significant decrease in the degree of epidermal hyperplasia/proliferation and the number of infiltrating dermal T cells, dendritic cells, and mast cells, and also they showed a reduction in TH2 and TH2-associated molecules. In a placebo-controlled, double-blind, phase 2 study in Japan, 79 adult patients with severe or very severe AD were randomized to ustekinumab 45 mg or 90 mg or placebo by subcutaneous injection at weeks 0 and 4. Neither of the 2 dosing regimens of ustekinumab resulted in significant improvement in the primary efficacy outcome of a percentage change in baseline Eczema Area and Severity Index (EASI) at week 12 versus placebo or improvement in major secondary efficacy end points.[39]

JANUS KINASE INHIBITORS

Janus kinase (JAK) signal transducer and activator of transcription (STAT) is a common intracellular signaling pathway for many proinflammatory cytokines involved in the pathophysiology of AD (eg, IL-4, IL-5, IL-13, IL-31).In mouse model studies of AD, JAK inhibitors have been shown to decrease IL-4, IL-5, IL-13, and IL-31 signaling and improve skin barrier functions. Various JAK inhibitors are being evaluated in early-phase human trials (listed in **Table 2**) for clinical efficacy. Tofacitinib is an oral small molecule JAK inhibitor approved for treatment of rheumatoid arthritis. Also, a topical formulation of tofacitinib has been shown to be beneficial for treatment of mild to moderate psoriasis. A phase II randomized trial of topical tofacitinib (2%) ointment used twice daily for 4 weeks showed significant improvement in EASI score in adults with mild to moderate AD compared with placebo.[40] Further trials of longer duration are needed, particularly because of the potential for immune suppression with JAK inhibitors.

Questions to Ask

As more new and promising therapeutics become available, some hard question need to be answered. Are these drugs likely to be effective in all patients with AD or only certain AD phenotypes? How to select a specific biologic agent for a patient? Are there any good biomarkers or clinical markers to guide therapy? What is the long-term safety and efficacy? What is the risk of severe reactions? What is the safety/efficacy of drugs in younger children in whom the disease is more prevalent? How long to treat, and what is the likelihood of relapse after the treatment is stopped? What is the impact on other comorbid allergic diseases, such as asthma? When will these drugs be available for clinical use, and how about coverage by insurance payers?

OTHER THERAPIES
Phototherapy

Phototherapy is an efficacious treatment of AD and has been shown to reduce levels of inflammatory cells in the skin, reverse epidermal hyperplasia, and reverse thickening of the stratum corneum, thereby improving the skin barrier to entry of external antigens, and also decreasing skin bacterial infections, particularly by S aureus.[20,41] Phototherapy can be given as monotherapy or in combination with other topical or systemic treatments. Narrow-band ultraviolet B is usually preferred in the United States for long-term or maintenance therapy for chronic AD because of its low-risk profile, relative efficacy, availability, and provider comfort. Short courses of ultraviolet A can be recommended for exacerbations and for patients with severe, widespread AD. The Joint Task Force and the American Academy of Dermatology have published guidance documents for phototherapy for AD.[20] Phototherapy is not approved for children younger than 12 years of age in the United States. Phototherapy is a specialized treatment and is usually available in larger health centers, thus accessibility is sometimes a problem. Tanning beds are not a safe alternative. The most common side effects are cutaneous, including actinic skin damage, erythema, pigmentary skin changes, and tenderness. Systemic effects such as cutaneous melanoma or nonmelanoma skin cancer, photosensitive eruptions, and cataract are less common.[20]

Systemic Immunomodulatory Agents

Systemic immunomodulatory agents are often considered in recalcitrant AD in both adult and pediatric patients unimproved with topical regimens and significant negative emotional and social impact.[20,42] Systemic corticosteroids are FDA approved to treat inflammatory skin disease, including severe, refractory AD, but only for a severe exacerbation and as a short-term bridge therapy, not for long-term daily maintenance treatment.[20] The risks of serious side effects, rebound of the disease when stopped, and hypothalamic-pituitary axis suppression outweigh any potential benefits.

Cyclosporine, methotrexate, azathioprine, and mycophenolate mofetil are all considered as off-label use for treatment of AD. Cyclosporine is a commonly preferred initial drug, followed by other drugs such as methotrexate or mycophenolate.[42] There are no consistent recommendations for dosing and treatment duration for these drugs because of insufficient data. Close monitoring for side effects and frequent blood testing are required.[20]

Anti–Immunoglobulin E Therapies

IgE is a hallmark of atopic disease and IgE levels are remarkably increased in patients with extrinsic AD. Anti-IgE treatment has been explored. A systemic review of 26 studies involving 174 patients using variable protocols of dosing study designs failed to show evidence to support omalizumab to treat AD.[43] The investigators suggested a subset of patients with AD, possibly those with an urticarial component to their disease, might still benefit from this therapy. Anti-IgE blockade with omalizumab has shown efficacy in treating other atopic diseases such as chronic idiopathic urticaria and moderate to severe allergic asthma. This finding suggests that increased IgE level is an epiphenomenon of AD, perhaps mediating comorbidities such as food allergies, allergic rhinoconjunctivitis, and asthma, but not contributing to symptoms and inflammation.

Allergen Immunotherapy

The Atopic Dermatitis Practice Parameter Update states that clinicians might consider allergen-specific immunotherapy (SIT) in selected patients with AD and aeroallergen sensitivity, but the data for this option are of limited quality.[44] SIT may be a treatment option for selected patients with proven sensitization to house dust and severe eczema that is not controlled with conventional therapies.

Probiotics, Prebiotics

Slow development of *Bifidobacterium* species and *Lactobacillus* species has been seen in the gut microflora of allergic children. Consumption of probiotics has been shown to stimulate intestinal microbiota and suppress the TH2 response, leading to improvements in the balance between TH1 and TH2. Probiotics, which are colonies of live microorganisms, or prebiotics, which are nondigestible oligosaccharides such as transgalactooligosaccharide and fructooligosaccharide, have been explored as prevention as well as for management of AD in many studies. A meta-analysis of 25 randomized controlled trials (n = 1599) studying the effectiveness of probiotics for treatment of AD were evaluated.[45] The primary outcome was significant differences in SCORAD (SCORing for Atopic Dermatitis) values favoring probiotics compared with the control. The significant value was seen in a group of children 1 to 18 years old (−5.74, 95% confidence interval−7.27 to −4.20), and in adults (−8.26, 95% confidence interval −13.28 to −3.25). However, the effectiveness of probiotics in infants (<1 year old) with AD was not proved. Treatment with a mixture of different bacterial species or of *Lactobacillus* species showed greater benefit than did treatment with *Bifidobacterium* species alone. Based on the review, the investigators suggested that probiotics could be an option for the treatment of AD, especially for moderate to severe AD in children and adults, but not in infants.[45] At this time, robust conclusions cannot be drawn, and more controlled studies are needed outlining dosage and species of probiotics benefiting patients with AD.

Cutaneous Microbiome

Patients with moderate to severe AD are associated with decreased diversity of skin microbiota and increased colonization of S aureus. S aureus obtained from severe AD skin has been shown to upregulate IL-4, IL-13, and Il-22 expressions and also induce epidermal thickening and expansion of TH2 and TH17 cells in a mouse model more than from patients with milder AD and healthy controls.[46] Commensal bacteria such as Staphylococcus epidermidis and Staphylococcus hominis seen on healthy skin have been shown to be protective against S aureus because of production of antimicrobial peptides and to decrease its colonization in patients with AD.[47] Anti–IL-4/IL-13 treatment (dupilumab) in phase II trials has also been shown to decrease S aureus in lesional and nonlesional skin and thus reduce infections more than placebo.[27,28] Therefore possible benefits of using commensal strains of coagulase-negative S epidermidis and S hominis from healthy donors applied to AD skin, or spraying the commensal gram-negative coccobacillus Roseomonas mucosa on the arms of patients with AD (NCT03018275, clinicaltrials.gov) or targeted transplant lotion of coagulase-negative staphylococci applied to the arms of adults with AD are being investigated (NCT03151148, clinicaltrials.gov).

Dietary Supplements/Chinese Herbal Medicines

Most studies, including meta-analyses, have failed to show a significant difference with active treatment using dietary supplements, including vitamins, fish oil, plant-derived essential fatty acids, primrose oil, and Chinese herbal medicines even though they have been used for long time as traditional remedies.[48,49]

Hospitalization/Multidisciplinary Approach

Some patients with severe AD are best served in a multidisciplinary clinic or even in day-hospital settings. Such facilities provide an opportunity for comprehensive education and hands-on demonstration of wet wraps, bathing/soaking, and topical treatments. This process may help identify triggers and stress, provide the services of nutritionists and behavioral therapists to address itch-scratch cycles and stress, and provide access to specialists including dermatologists and allergists in a single platform to improve outcomes.[50]

SUMMARY

AD is a complex systemic inflammatory disease. Long-standing topical therapies are not sufficient for treating severe AD or to improve quality of life. Systemic immunomodulating agents are limited by side effects and by their effectiveness. Targeted new therapies promise to be more effective and to maintain improvement with fewer side effects.

REFERENCES

1. Simpson EL, Irvine ADM, Eichenfield LFM, et al. Update on epidemiology, diagnosis, and disease course of atopic dermatitis. Semin Cutan Med Surg 2016;35: S84–8.

2. Schneider L, Tilles S, Lio P, et al. Atopic dermatitis: a practice parameter update 2012. J Allergy Clin Immunol 2013;131:295–9.e1-27.

3. Carroll CL, Balkrishnan R, Feldman SR, et al. The burden of atopic dermatitis: impact on the patients, family, and society. Pediatr Dermatol 2005;22:192–9.

4. Narla S, Silverberg JI. Association between atopic dermatitis and serious cutaneous, multiorgan and systemic infections in US adults. Ann Allergy Asthma Immunol 2018;120:66–72.

5. Brunner PM, Silverberg JI, Guttman-Yassky E, et al. Increasing comorbidities suggest that atopic dermatitis is a systemic disorder. J Invest Dermatol 2017; 137:18–25.

6. Boginiewicz M, Leung DY. Atopic dermatitis: a disease of altered skin barrier and immune dysregulation. Immunol Rev 2011;242:233–46.

7. Czarnowicki T, Krueger JG, Guttman-Yassky E. Skin barrier and immune dysregulation in atopic dermatitis: an evolving story with important clinical implications. J Allergy Clin Immunol Pract 2014;2:371–9.

8. Werfel T, Allam JP, Biedermann T, et al. Cellular and molecular immunologic mechanisms in patients with atopic dermatitis. J Allergy Clin Immunol 2016; 138:336–49.

9. Czarnowicki T, Krueger JG, Guttman-Yassky E. Novel concepts of prevention and treatment of atopic dermatitis through barrier and immune manipulations with implications for the atopic march. J Allergy Clin Immunol 2017;139:1723e–34e.

10. Sehra S, Yao Y, Howell MD, et al. IL-4 regulates skin homeostasis and the predisposition toward allergic skin inflammation. J Immunol 2010;184:3186–90.

11. Kisich KO, Carspecken CW, Fieve S, et al. Defective killing of Staphylococcus aureus in atopic dermatitis is associated with reduced mobilization of human beta-defensin-3. J Allergy Clin Immunol 2008;122:62–8.

12. Eyerich K, Pennino D, Scarponi C, et al. IL-17 in atopic eczema: linking allergen-specific adaptive and microbial-triggered innate immune response. J Allergy Clin Immunol 2009;123:59–66.

13. Akdis CA, Akdis M. Immunological differences between intrinsic and extrinsic types of atopic dermatitis. Clin Exp Allergy 2003;33:1618–21, ena GA, Vestita M, Cassano N.

14. Shi B, Bangayan NJ, Curd E, et al. The skin microbiome is different in pediatric versus adult atopic dermatitis. J Allergy Clin Immunol 2016;138:1233–6.

15. Esaki H, Brunner PM, Renert-Yuval Y, et al. Early-onset pediatric atopic dermatitis is TH2 but also TH17 polarized in skin. J Allergy Clin Immunol 2016;138:1639e–51e.

16. Noda S, Suarez-Farinas M, Ungar B, et al. The Asian atopic dermatitis phenotype combines features of atopic dermatitis and psoriasis with increased TH17 polarization. J Allergy Clin Immunol 2015;136:1254–64.

17. Margolis DJ, Apter AJ, Gupta J, et al. The persistence of atopic dermatitis and filaggrin (FLG) mutations in a US longitudinal cohort. J Allergy Clin Immunol 2012;130:912–7.

18. Eichenfield LF, Tom WL, Chamlin SL, et al. Guidelines of care for the management of atopic dermatitis: section 1.Diagnosis and assessment of atopic dermatitis. J Am Acad Dermatol 2014;70:338–51.

19. Eichenfield LF, Tom WL, Berger TG, et al. Guidelines of care for the management of atopic dermatitis: section 2. Management and treatment of atopic dermatitis with topical therapies. J Am Acad Dermatol 2014;71:116–32.

20. Sidbury R, Davis DM, Cohen DE, et al. Guidelines of care for the management of atopic dermatitis: section 3. Management and treatment with phototherapy and systemic agents. J Am Acad Dermatol 2014;71:327–49.

21. Sidbury R, Tom WL, Bergman JN, et al. Guidelines of care for the management of atopic dermatitis: section 4. Prevention of disease flares and use of adjunctive therapies and approaches. J Am Acad Dermatol 2014;71:1218–33.

22. Hanifin JM, Chan SC, Cheng JB, et al. Type 4 phosphodiesterase inhibitors have clinical and in vitro anti-inflammatory effects in atopic dermatitis. J Invest Dermatol 1996;107:51–6.

23. Paller AS, Tom WL, Lebwohl MG, et al. Efficacy and safety of crisaborole ointment, a novel, nonsteroidal phosphodiesterase 4 (PDE4) inhibitor for the topical treatment of atopic dermatitis (AD) in children and adults. J Am Acad Dermatol 2016;75:494–503.

24. Zane LT, Chanda S, Jarnagin K, et al. Crisaborole and its potential role in treating atopic dermatitis: overview of early clinical studies. Immunotherapy 2016;8: 853–66.

25. Paller AS, Kabashima K, Thomas B. Therapeutic pipeline for atopic dermatitis: End of the drought? J Allergy Clin Immunol 2017;140(3):633–43.

26. Beck LA, Thaci D, Hamilton JD, et al. Dupilumab treatment in adults with moderate-to severe atopic dermatitis. N Engl J Med 2014;371:130–9.

27. Simpson EL, Bieber T, Guttman-Yassky E, et al. Two phase 3 trials of dupilumab versus placebo in atopic dermatitis. N Engl J Med 2016;375:2335–48.

28. Blauvelt A, de Bruin-Weller M, Gooderham M, et al. Long-term management of moderate-to-severe atopic dermatitis with dupilumab and concomitant topical corticosteroids (LIBERTY AD CHRONOS): a 1-year, randomised, double-blinded, placebo-controlled, phase 3 trial. Lancet 2017;389:2287–303.

29. Busse WW, Maspero JF, Rabe KF, et al. Liberty Asthma QUEST: Phase 3 Randomized, Double-Blind, Placebo-Controlled, Parallel-Group Study to Evaluate Dupilumab Efficacy/Safety in Patients with Uncontrolled, Moderate-to-Severe Asthma. Adv Ther 2018. https://doi.org/10.1007/s12325-018-0702-4.

30. Dupixent® (dupilumab) injection, for subcutaneous use [prescribing information]. Bridgewater (NJ): Regeneron Pharmaceuticals, Sanofi-Aventis US, LLC; 2017.

31. Wollenberg A, Howell MD, Guttman-Yassky E, et al. A phase 2b dose-ranging efficacy and safety study of tralokinumab in adult patients with moderate to severe atopic dermatitis (AD). Presented at the Annual Meeting of the American Academy of Dermatology; 2017.

32. Simpson EL, Flohr C, Eichenfield L. Efficacy and safety of lebrikizumab in patients with atopic dermatitis: a phase II randomized, controlled trial (TREBLE). Presented at the 25th Congress of the European Academy of Dermatology and Venerology; 2016.

33. Oldhoff JM, Darsow U, Werfel T, et al. Anti IL-5 recombinant humanized monoclonal antibody (mepolizumab) for the treatment of atopic dermatitis. Allergy 2005;60:693e–6e.

34. Kato A, Fujii E, Watanabe T, et al. Distribution of IL-31 and its receptor expressing cells in skin of atopic dermatitis. J Dermatol Sci 2014;74:229–35.

35. Ruzicka T, Hanifin JM, Furue M, et al. Anti interleukin-31 receptor a antibody for atopic dermatitis. N Engl J Med 2017;376:826e835.

36. Kabashima K, Furue M, Hanifin JM, et al. Nemolizumab in patients with moderate-to-severe atopic dermatitis: Randomized, phase II, long-term extension study. J Allergy Clin Immunol 2018;142:1121–30.

37. Guttman-Yassky E, Khattri S, Brunner PM, et al. A pathogenic role for Th22/IL-22 in atopic dermatitis is established by a placebo-controlled trial with an anti-IL-22/ILV-094 mAb[abstract]. J Invest Dermatol 2017;137(suppl):S53.

38. Weiss D, Schaschinger M, Ristl R, et al. Ustekinumab treatment in severe atopic dermatitis: down-regulation of T-helper 2/22 expression. J Am Acad Dermatol 2017;76:91–7.e3.

39. Saeki H, Kabashima K, Tokura Y, et al. Efficacy and safety of ustekinumab in Japanese patients with severe atopic dermatitis: a randomised, double-blind, placebo-controlled, phase II Study. Br J Dermatol 2017;177:419–27.
40. Bissonnette R, Papp KA, Poulin Y, et al. Topical tofacitinib for atopic dermatitis: a phase IIa randomized trial. Br J Dermatol 2016;175:902–11.
41. Patrizi A, Raone B, Ravaioli GM. Management of atopic dermatitis: safety and efficacy of phototherapy. Clin Cosmet Investig Dermatol 2015;8:511–20.
42. Roekevisch E, Spuls PI, Kuester D, et al. Efficacy and safety of systemic treatments for moderate-to-severe atopic dermatitis: a systematic review. J Allergy Clin Immunol 2014;133:429–38.
43. Wang H-H, Li Y-C, Huang Y-C. Efficacy of omalizumab in patients with atopic dermatitis: a systematic review and meta-analysis. J Allergy Clin Immunol 2016;138:1719–22.
44. Bae JM, Choi YY, Park CO, et al. Efficacy of allergen-specific immunotherapy for atopic dermatitis: a systematic review and meta-analysis of randomized controlled trials. J Allergy Clin Immunol 2013;132:110.
45. Kim S-O, Ah Y-M, Yu YM, et al. Effects of probiotics for the treatment of atopic dermatitis: a meta-analysis of randomized controlled trials. Ann Allergy Asthma Immunol 2014;113:217–26.
46. Byrd AL, Deming C, Cassidy SKB, et al. Staphylococcus aureus and Staphylococcus epidermidis strain diversity underlying pediatric atopic dermatitis. Sci Transl Med 2017;9(397) [pii:eaal4651].
47. Nakatsuji T, Chen TH, Narala S, et al. Antimicrobials from human skin commensal bacteria protect against Staphylococcus aureus and are deficient in atopic dermatitis. Sci Transl Med 2017;9(378) [pii: eaah4680]. Systemic immunomodulating drugs.
48. Bath-Hextall FJ, Jenkinson C, Humphreys R, et al. Dietary supplements for established atopic eczema. Cochrane Database Syst Rev 2012;(2):CD005205.
49. Koo J, Arain S. Traditional Chinese medicine for the treatment of dermatologic disorders. Arch Dermatol 1998;134:1388.
50. LeBovidge JS, Elverson W, Timmons KG, et al. Multidisciplinary interventions in the management of atopic dermatitis. J Allergy Clin Immunol 2016;138:325–34.

Pediatric Drug Allergies

Updates on Beta-Lactam, Nonsteroidal Anti-Inflammatory Drug, and Chemotherapeutic Reactions

Shazia Lutfeali, MD, David A. Khan, MD*

KEYWORDS

- Pediatric drug allergies • Hypersensitivity reactions • Beta lactam antibiotics
- Non-beta lactam antibiotics • Nonsteroidal anti-inflammatory drugs
- Chemotherapeutics

KEY POINTS

- Beta-lactam antibiotics and nonsteroidal anti-inflammatory drugs remain the most common causes of pediatric drug hypersensitivity, although only a minority of reactions is generally confirmed as true drug allergy.
- Diagnosis typically requires drug challenges because of the lack of standardized and widely available in vivo and in vitro testing.
- An understanding of pediatric drug allergies as well as methods to diagnose true drug allergies is important.

INTRODUCTION

Adverse drug reactions are frequently reported in pediatric patients. A 2012 systematic review found that the overall incidence of adverse drug reactions reached up to 16.8% in hospitalized children and up to 11.0% in outpatient children.[1] Drug allergic reactions account for a lower percentage of all adverse drug reactions, and after evaluation only a minority of presumed drug allergy is confirmed as true drug allergy.[2,3] For instance, penicillin allergy testing performed in pediatric populations successfully removes penicillin allergy labels from about 96% of patients.[4] Drug allergy labels in children are associated with adverse clinical outcomes; specifically, antibiotic allergy labels correlate with significant alternate antibiotic use and longer hospital stays.[5] Therefore, an understanding of pediatric drug allergies as well as methods to diagnose true drug allergies is important. In this review article, the authors discuss pediatric drug allergies

Department of Internal Medicine, Division of Allergy & Immunology, The University of Texas Southwestern Medical Center, 5323 Harry Hines Boulevard, Dallas, TX 75390-8859, USA
* Corresponding author.
E-mail address: dave.khan@utsouthwestern.edu

Pediatr Clin N Am 66 (2019) 1035–1051
https://doi.org/10.1016/j.pcl.2019.06.006
0031-3955/19/© 2019 Elsevier Inc. All rights reserved.

with emphasis on the most common culprits, beta-lactam (BL) antibiotics and nonsteroidal anti-inflammatory drugs (NSAIDs). Also included are brief sections on desensitization considerations.

In the pediatric population, BL antibiotics are the most commonly involved drug group followed by NSAIDs and non-BL antibiotics.

PREVALENCE

The most common drugs implicated in pediatric drug hypersensitivity reactions are BL antibiotics and NSAIDs, followed by non-BL antibiotics. As in adults, the most common manifestations are cutaneous, although true drug hypersensitivity is less likely to be confirmed in pediatric than in adult patients.[6–8] In addition, although drug reactions are more common in adult women than men,[9] in children, the gender distribution seems approximately equal.[2,5] Of note, the occurrence of pathogen-induced cutaneous symptoms, which may be mistaken for drug reaction, is an important consideration. A 2011 study of children presenting to the emergency department with maculopapular or urticarial rash in the setting of BL antibiotic use found that when later challenged to the culprit drug, only 6.8% of children had reproducible rash. Most children resulted positive for viral studies, highlighting the relevance of viral exanthem in these situations.[10] There is also a known association of rash in the setting of amoxicillin administration during Epstein-Barr virus (EBV) infection. Interestingly, however, a recent study showed that of the 18.6% of EBV-infected patients who developed rash, approximately half were treated with antibiotics, implying that EBV-associated rash in the setting of antibiotic use may be less common than previously thought.[11]

CHARACTERIZATION OF HYPERSENSITIVITY

Drug allergic reactions in general can be classified as immediate or nonimmediate. Immediate reactions usually occur within 1 hour of drug intake (but may occur up to 6 hours after drug exposure) and are typically mediated by immunoglobulin E (IgE) antibodies; they commonly present as urticaria or anaphylaxis.[12] Nonimmediate reactions usually occur days later (but can occur earlier) and are typically T cell mediated. They may present as maculopapular, delayed onset urticaria, other rashes, or rarely, as a severe cutaneous adverse reaction (SCAR). The immunopathogenesis of SCAR is complex and is beyond the scope of this review but has been recently reviewed elsewhere.[13]

PENICILLIN AND OTHER BETA-LACTAM ANTIBIOTICS

Traditionally, diagnostic guidelines for addressing penicillin allergy have been similar in children and adults. However, given the difficulty of adhering to these protocols in children (ie, time required for testing, painful intradermal injections), the benign and typically delayed nature of most reactions,[3] the natural history of waning antibiotic sensitivity over time,[14] and consideration that diagnostic protocols in adults may not have equal diagnostic accuracy in children, recent studies have addressed the utility of standard protocols with skin testing versus direct antibiotic challenge, particularly in low-risk patients.

Single-Day Challenge

Although several smaller studies in children had previously evaluated the role of direct drug challenge without skin testing in children, the first large prospective study was conducted by Mill and colleagues.[15] They performed a prospective study of 818 children with histories of suspected amoxicillin allergy. Only children with SCAR were excluded. Children with anaphylaxis were not excluded, but none were enrolled. All children underwent a graded oral challenge with 10% of the therapeutic dose of amoxicillin followed 20 minutes later by 90% of the therapeutic dose and were observed for at least 1 hour. Among the 818 children challenged with amoxicillin, 94.1% tolerated the challenge with 2.1% having immediate (<1 hour) reactions and 3.8% having delayed reactions. Immediate reactions occurred in 17 children, were all mild, and consisted of hives only. Skin testing was performed 2 to 3 months later and only 1 of 17 had a positive penicillin skin test. In addition, children with histories of serum sickness-like reactions also safely underwent challenge using this protocol with no severe reactions occurring.

Ibanez and colleagues[16] subsequently assessed penicillin allergy in 732 children with histories of nonsevere reactions. Drug provocation tests were administered regardless of skin testing and serum-specific IgE results. Only 4.8% of patients were found to be penicillin allergic, compared with higher rates of penicillin allergy (7.9%–16.7%) in prior studies in which drug provocation tests were only performed in cases of negative skin and serum-specific IgE testing.[6,17,18] The investigators concluded that penicillin protocols, which have known accuracy in adults,[9] may not be equally diagnostic in children and may actually result in overdiagnosis. High specificity and low sensitivity for intradermal and specific IgE testing were seen; specificity for intradermal testing and specific IgE resulted at 98.3% and 99%, respectively, whereas sensitivity resulted very low at 9.1% and 2.9%. Interestingly, none of the 5.2% of patients with histories of immediate index reactions were shown to have true penicillin allergy via drug provocation test. Also of note, cefuroxime was tolerated by all but one of the penicillin-allergic patients who were administered cefuroxime challenge.

Confino-Cohen and colleagues[19] evaluated direct challenge in 642 patients with histories of nonimmediate reactions, which included 435 children. They also performed skin tests and drug provocation regardless of test results. Despite a relatively high rate of positive or equivocal skin tests (5.2% and 32.4%), 96.1% of these patients tolerated the first day graded challenge. **Table 1** summarizes these studies.

Table 1			
Penicillin challenge studies without prior skin testing, or regardless of skin testing results			
Penicillin Direct Challenge Studies		**Penicillin Extended Challenge Studies**	
Study	**Outcomes**	**Study**	**Outcomes**
Mill et al,[15] 2016	Of 818 pediatric patients, 5.9% developed mild reactions	Mori et al,[20] 2015	Of 200 pediatric patients given 5-d provocation tests, 9.6% developed reactions
Confino-Cohen et al,[19] 2017[a]	Of 617 pediatric patients, 5.3% developed reactions	Vezir et al,[21] 2016	Of 119 pediatric patients given 5-d provocation tests, 3.4% developed urticarial reactions
Ibanez et al,[16] 2018	Of 732 pediatric patients, 4.8% developed nonsevere reactions	Confino-Cohen et al,[19] 2017[a]	Of 491 pediatric patients given complete/partial 5-d provocation tests, 6.1% developed mild reactions
Iammatteo et al,[22] 2018	Of 155 patients ≥7 y old, 2.6% developed mild reactions	Labrosse et al,[23] 2018	Of 130 patients given 5-d provocation tests, 6.2% developed positive/equivocal reactions

Most studies enrolled patients with non-severe reactions histories.
[a] References the same study.

Prolonged Challenge

Despite the delayed nature of most pediatric BL reactions, delayed intradermal testing and patch testing have been shown to be of limited diagnostic utility.[6,24] A few studies have addressed the value of prolonged oral provocation challenge in diagnosing non-immediate BL hypersensitivity (see **Table 1**).

Mori and colleagues[20] showed an increase in detection of nonimmediate reactions from 35.7% to 100% with use of prolonged 5-day challenges in a European pediatric cohort of 200 patients with suspected amoxicillin allergy. In the aforementioned study by Confino-Cohen and colleagues,[19] they also found increased detection of nonimmediate reactions; an additional 6.1% of cohort patients developed mild delayed reactions during prolonged 5-day challenge compared with 1-day challenge. No significant correlation was seen with skin testing results, and the investigators concluded that the penicillin allergy label could safely be removed using supervised graded challenge followed by ambulatory prolonged 5-day total oral challenge, without preceding skin test.

Recently, Labrosse and colleagues[23] assessed safety and efficacy of the 5-day challenge in diagnosing BL allergy and also implications for future BL antibiotic use. One hundred thirty Canadian participants with histories of nonsevere reactions (most of which were delayed) underwent blinded skin testing and graded drug provocation challenge with amoxicillin, regardless of skin testing results. Those patients with initial challenges underwent home amoxicillin administration for a total 5-day course. Patients who were ultimately diagnosed as nonallergic were contacted 2 years later to assess subsequent amoxicillin usage and tolerance, and data were compared with a prior similar group who had received a single-dose graded drug provocation challenge with oral penicillin. Of the study participants, 3 patients had a positive immediate challenge, 3 patients had a positive nonimmediate challenge (all of which were mild cutaneous reactions, suggesting safety of this ambulatory approach), and 2 were equivocal. Of note, parental anxiety was also assessed, and it was determined that almost half of the parents had been very or extremely frightened by their child's initial allergic reaction. Overall, the 5-day drug provocation test resulted in a significant 24.1% decrease in future penicillin avoidance compared with classical single-dose drug provocation challenge performed for 1 day in the historical cohort. The investigators concluded that 5-day challenge ensures better compliance with future penicillin use.

Discussion

Overall, these recent data specific to amoxicillin or penicillin allergy in children suggest that direct provocation without preceding skin testing appears to be safe and effective. This approach has not been evaluated for those rare children with anaphylactic reactions. Whether prolonged challenges are necessary is still a matter of debate. The length of prolonged challenge (5 days) appears reasonable, because prior studies have reported mean reaction delays of 3.8 days and 5.8 days.[6,24] However, as previously discussed, these reactions tend to be benign, and it is unclear whether accurately diagnosing a small additional percentage of patients with delayed drug hypersensitivity warrants subjecting all patients to prolonged antibiotic courses, with potential adverse effects. In an era of antimicrobial stewardship, full therapeutic courses of antibiotics without need are problematic. In addition, reactions elicited during prolonged challenges may in fact be due to delayed reactions after the first dose. Garcia Rodriguez and colleagues[25] recently proposed a modified protocol in which subjects underwent supervised challenge followed by a home observation period of at least the time elapsed between first dose and symptoms of the index reaction. Children who did not develop a reaction continued with prolonged ambulatory challenge. Alternatively, adequate cumulative dose may be more relevant than the timing of exposure.

Although prolonged challenges do appear to increase future use of penicillin antibiotics, which is ultimately the goal of addressing penicillin allergies, the main reason to adopt this approach seems to be for parental and provider reassurance. For instance, 1 study showed that even after their children had undergone negative penicillin skin testing and drug challenge, 18% of parents still refused penicillin-class antibiotics because of fear of adverse reaction.[26] It remains to be seen whether this objective can be accomplished to the same extent in the pediatric population via better education and effective interventions.

SPECIAL CONSIDERATIONS

Children with cystic fibrosis are generally thought to have a higher prevalence of hypersensitivity reactions to one or more antibiotics, especially BLs, which may be due in part to frequent exposure.[27] At least 1 study, though, has shown the opposite finding.[28]

DESENSITIZATION CONSIDERATIONS

Desensitization is defined as temporary induction of tolerance that can be maintained by continuous exposure to the medication. In the case of penicillin and BL allergy, desensitization is an option in those with histories of immediate reactions and positive skin tests and/or drug provocations. Desensitization may be considered when no alternative treatment exists for optimal therapy, and published data for BL and other antibiotic desensitizations in children largely involve the cystic fibrosis population. In general, proposed desensitization protocols for pediatric patients are similar to those used in adults but differ in the final dose administered. When possible, the oral route is preferred, and one of the most widely used protocols for penicillin has been published by Sullivan and colleagues.[29,30] IV protocols are also available[31] and can be adapted for pediatric patients. Successful desensitization to nonpenicillin BL antibiotics has also been performed.[32]

NONSTEROIDAL ANTI-INFLAMMATORY DRUGS

NSAIDs are the other common cause of pediatric drug hypersensitivity.[33] Along with antibiotics, NSAIDs account for most adverse drug reactions among outpatient children.[1] Similarly to antibiotics, NSAID hypersensitivity is less likely to be confirmed in children than adults, and viral infections are an important confounding factor.[34] Recent studies have shown rates of 16.9% to 24% of confirmed NSAID hypersensitivity via drug challenge,[35,36] although prior studies have reported higher rates. Unlike adult patients with NSAID hypersensitivity, in younger children, boys are as frequently if not more frequently involved.[36,37]

Classifications and Hypersensitivity Mechanisms

NSAIDs can induce hypersensitivity reactions via immunologic and nonimmunologic mechanisms (**Table 2**). In general, reactions are classified as selective to a particular drug or NSAID subclass or nonselective (cross-intolerant). Of these, the nonselective reactions are more frequent. One study showed a distribution of 58% nonselective reactions and 42% selective reactions in children; ibuprofen was the culprit drug in most

Table 2
Hypersensitivity reactions to nonsteroidal anti-inflammatory drugs

	Hypersensitivity Reactions to NSAIDs	
	Selective (Cross-Tolerant)	Nonselective (Cross-Intolerant)
Type of reaction	Single NSAID-induced urticaria/ angioedema or anaphylaxis	NERD
	Single NSAID-induced delayed hypersensitivity reaction	NECD
		Multiple NSAID-induced urticaria and angioedema
Possible mechanism of action	IgE mediated (immediate) or T-cell mediated (delayed)	COX-1 inhibition
Skin testing useful?	Limited to no data available, except for propyphenazone	No

of both nonselective and selective reactions.[38] Atopy and older age at first reaction are recognized risk factors for NSAID hypersensitivity.[35]

Nonselective or cross-intolerant reactions are triggered by more than 1 subclass of NSAIDs and encompass NSAID-exacerbated respiratory disease (NERD), NSAID-exacerbated cutaneous disease (NECD) in patients with chronic idiopathic urticaria, and multiple NSAID-induced urticaria and angioedema in otherwise healthy patients.[39] The latter commonly presents as isolated periorbital edema in children. Nonselective reactions occur when COX-1 inhibition plus an intrinsic defect in arachidonic acid metabolism leads to leukotriene generation and release of mast-cell and eosinophil-derived mediators.[33] Selective NSAID hypersensitivity reactions may be immediate or delayed. Immediate reactions are most likely mediated by specific IgE antibody, although identification of these antibodies is difficult via either skin testing or specific IgE assays with the exception of the NSAID propyphenazone, whereby positive skin tests and specific IgE have been reported in most of the studied individuals.[40] Selective delayed-type reactions are likely due to specific T-cell responses and can manifest in a variety of ways, including cutaneous reactions (eg, fixed drug eruptions), aseptic meningitis, and pneumonitis. Not all patients fit easily into these criteria and are often referred to as having a blended or mixed reaction as one that does not strictly meet criteria outlined by the aforementioned classification.[39]

The need for a pediatric-specific classification guideline for NSAID hypersensitivity reactions has been recognized. Cousin and colleagues[35] attempted to classify 635 pediatric patients with confirmed NSAID hypersensitivity according to the European Network on Drug Allergy (ENDA) classification, which does not differentiate between age groups. They found that 44% of patients did not fall strictly into 1 of the 5 categories outlined by the ENDA, and that no patient exhibited features strictly corresponding to NERD. The ENDA/European Academy of Allergy and Clinical Immunology recently released a consensus document with a proposed pediatric classification with distinct criteria for children younger than 10 years and 10 years of age to adolescence. The classification attempts to emphasize differences between NSAID hypersensitivity reactions between different age groups, with reactions in younger children typically being nonimmunologic, nonselective, and frequently occurring in the setting of confounding factors, such as viral illnesses. The proposed classification for older children is similar to the adult classification and takes into account the importance of anaphylactic reactions in this age group.[33]

Diagnosis

Diagnosis of NSAID-induced hypersensitivity is often difficult for several reasons, including presence of confounding factors (such as infection or concurrent use of other drugs), lack of established in vivo or in vitro diagnostic methods, and unclear natural history of NSAID allergy and effect of age.[33] As with antibiotics, the gold standard for diagnosis is the drug provocation test. Protocols vary based on the type of reaction to NSAIDs. Skin testing is not considered useful in nonselective reactions, because of the nonimmunologic nature of these reactions. There are also little to no data on skin testing with selective NSAID-induced delayed reactions. As mentioned previously, skin testing may be useful for reactions to propyphenazone. In contrast, most children skin tested with metamizole are negative.[41,42] However, at this time, skin testing is not recommended for most common NSAIDs because nonirritating concentrations are unknown, there is a lack of parenteral agents, and negative predictive values have not yet been established. In vitro studies are not widely available, and their diagnostic and predictive values also have yet to be validated, particularly in children.[43]

Nonselective Reactions and Tolerance of Alternative Agents

Although the natural history of nonselective reactions is unknown, it is thought that some patients may develop tolerance over time, especially patients with chronic urticaria because chronic urticaria remits. Therefore, periodic reevaluation is warranted. Acetaminophen/paracetamol at standard doses is generally considered safe in patients with nonselective reactions, although drug challenge may be advisable.[38] One study looked at the incidence of aspirin hypersensitivity (using a maximum cumulative dose of 500 mg aspirin) in children and adolescents with chronic urticaria, which was found to be 22%. All patients were able to tolerate acetaminophen/paracetamol.[44] Another study found that all participants with confirmed COX-1 inhibitor hypersensitivity, diagnosed via drug challenge to aspirin and the culprit NSAID, were able to tolerate acetaminophen/paracetamol as well as etoricoxib, a selective COX-2 inhibitor. Most study participants were able to tolerate meloxicam, a preferential COX-2 inhibitor.[37,45]

Special Considerations

In general, use of NSAIDs has been correlated with asthma exacerbations in children. Lo and colleagues[46] showed an association between short-term use of ibuprofen, aspirin, and diclofenac and increased rates of asthma exacerbations resulting in asthma-related hospitalizations. Debley and colleagues[47] found a prevalence rate of 2% ibuprofen-sensitive asthma in a study of school-aged children with mild to moderate asthma. NSAIDs have also been implicated in the occurrence of food-associated and/or exercise-induced anaphylaxis, more so in adolescents.[48]

Desensitization Considerations

In adults, aspirin-exacerbated respiratory disease (AERD)/NERD is one of the primary indications for aspirin desensitization. This condition rarely manifests before the third decade of life; however, there have been case reports as well as a small study with children as young as 8 years old and adolescents diagnosed with AERD/NERD.[49–51] In 1 report, a 16-year-old female adolescent with recurrent polyps underwent aspirin desensitization as per the adult protocol proposed by Lee and Stevenson[45] and experienced long-term clinical benefit on a daily 300-mg dose of aspirin.[50] In another report, an 8 year-old girl and a 12-year-old girl underwent successful aspirin desensitization via intranasal ketorolac challenge and desensitization followed by aspirin desensitization and ultimately tolerated 650 mg aspirin twice daily, although aspirin was subsequently discontinued in the younger patient owing to debilitating urticaria.[51,52] As the pediatric AERD/NERD population has recently been recognized, the efficacy of high-dose aspirin in these patients has not been investigated. Aspirin is generally avoided in pediatrics because of concern for Reye syndrome; the chief exception is Kawasaki disease, which typically presents in young children. Review of the literature does not reveal cases of Kawasaki disease in which aspirin desensitization was necessary. In cases of pain or inflammatory conditions in which NSAIDs/acetylsalicylic acid are not tolerated, it appears that alternative agents are frequently used.

NON–BETA-LACTAM ANTIBIOTICS

Hypersensitivity reactions to non-BL antibiotics, such as aminoglycosides, fluoroquinolones, and macrolides, are rare compared with BL antibiotics. Diagnosis of IgE-mediated allergy to these drugs is difficult due to limited knowledge about relevant metabolites and allergenic determinants. Nonirritating skin test concentrations have been published, but for the most part have not yet been validated in children.[53–55] In addition, the negative predictive values for these tests is unknown. In general, non-BL antibiotics are uncommon causes of anaphylactic reactions.[54]

Most pediatric studies on non-BL antibiotics consist of case reports or small series of patients.[55] Guvenir and colleagues[56] recently addressed hypersensitivity to non-BL antibiotics in children using intradermal concentrations that have previously been published in adults; of the 85 patients with nonsevere reaction histories who underwent testing, non-BL hypersensitivity was confirmed in 4.7%. Those patients with a history of anaphylactic reactions or recent antihistamine ingestion underwent desensitization in lieu of testing.

SULFONAMIDE ANTIBIOTICS

In general, reactions to sulfonamides rarely manifest as IgE-mediated reactions and more frequently present as delayed hypersensitivity reactions, some of which can be life-threatening SCARs, such as Stevens-Johnson syndrome (SJS), toxic epidermal necrolysis (TEN), and drug reaction with eosinophilia and systemic symptoms (DRESS).[9] A pooled analysis of 2 multicenter case-control studies showed that sulfonamide antibiotics were identified as 1 of 4 drugs most commonly associated with SJS/TEN in patients less than 15 years of age.[57] Skin testing with nonirritating concentrations can be used for immediate reactions, and delayed intradermal testing and/or patch testing can be used for nonimmediate reactions.[55,56] The drug provocation test is the gold standard for diagnosis but is contraindicated in patients with severe reaction histories.[55] Although alternate therapy is preferred, continuation of therapy ("treating through") with or without addition of antihistamines, steroids, or other medications may be an option for those who require sulfonamide therapy (eg, those with human immunodeficiency virus [HIV] and *Pneumocystis jirovecii* pneumonia) and have a history of mild cutaneous eruptions without mucosal involvement.[58] The role of desensitization in non-IgE-mediated reactions is unclear. Numerous reports of successful desensitizations for sulfonamide antibiotics exist, including in pediatric patients, particularly those with HIV.[59,60] However, studies in adults comparing drug reaction rates immediately following sulfonamide drug provocation versus drug desensitizations have shown similar tolerability.[61–63]

MACROLIDES

In general, hypersensitivity reactions to macrolides are reported less frequently than sulfonamides.[55] In a study of adult and pediatric patients with a history of macrolide hypersensitivity, none of the confirmed reactions occurred in pediatric patients.[64] Clarithromycin is probably the best studied; the rate of confirmed hypersensitivity in children is low and may range from 2.1% to 6%.[56,65] Skin testing to clarithromycin has shown variable reliability, and different studies have used different nonirritating concentrations.[65] Based on this, many experts do not recommend skin testing for evaluation of macrolide allergy.[66] Anaphylaxis to macrolides has traditionally been considered very rare; however, a recent study showed a somewhat higher anaphylaxis rate of 4.5%.[67] Cross-reactivity can occur between different macrolides.[67,68] A case of successful desensitization to clarithromycin in a pediatric patient has been reported.[69]

AMINOGLYCOSIDES

Aminoglycoside use occurs more so in the newborn and cystic fibrosis populations than in healthy children. In general, anaphylaxis in the neonatal period is uncommon; however, a case report of anaphylaxis to amikacin in a premature newborn has been reported.[70] Neomycin is a recognized contact allergen, and patch tests with neomycin have been shown to be positive in 5% of children with contact dermatitis less than 3 years of age.[71] Overall, however, aminoglycoside hypersensitivity is uncommon, but immediate reactions can be evaluated by skin testing. Cross-reactivity between different aminoglycoside antibiotics has been shown to occur.[72] Desensitization, particularly in cystic fibrosis patients, has been performed successfully.[72–74]

FLUOROQUINOLONES

Historically, fluoroquinolone use in pediatrics has been avoided because of concern for adverse effects, although fluoroquinolone prescription rates have increased in recent years.[75] In adults, frequency of immediate reactions to quinolones appear to be increasing, possibly because of increased use of these antibiotics, and it is likely that the same trend will manifest in pediatrics.[9] Use of fluoroquinolones is particularly relevant in the cystic fibrosis population; desensitization has been performed in children with and without cystic fibrosis.[76,77] Patients with allergy to 1 fluoroquinolone antibiotic may be able to tolerate another, and there are no clear patterns of cross-reactivity.[78]

CHEMOTHERAPEUTICS

Hypersensitivity reactions have been reported with almost all chemotherapeutic agents.[79–81] Diagnosing hypersensitivity to chemotherapeutics is challenging, because patients receiving these agents are frequently immunocompromised, are administered multiple medications simultaneously, and have symptom overlap with infusion reactions, chemotherapy toxicity, or graft-versus-host disease.[82] In particular, cutaneous eruptions occur commonly in children receiving chemotherapy; for example, Lim and colleagues[83] recently reported a case of flagellate dermatitis in a child most likely from doxorubicin. Another phenomenon reported by Webber and colleagues[82] was described as a distinct, self-limited intertriginous eruption, which was not associated with a particular malignancy or medication but was associated with high-dose chemotherapy regimens. Of note, corticosteroids, often used in the treatment of hypersensitivity reactions, must be used with caution in the oncology population. For instance, pediatric patients with acute myelogenous leukemia have an increased risk of death associated with corticosteroid administration.[79] This discussion focuses on select chemotherapeutic agents, which more commonly cause hypersensitivity reactions in children and those for which desensitizations have been performed. The 3-solution, 12-step protocol published by Castells and colleagues[84] has been shown to be widely applicable to multiple medications, with similar protocols currently being used in pediatric patients.[85]

PLATINUM-BASED DRUGS (CISPLATIN, CARBOPLATIN, OXALIPLATIN)

Carboplatin is used for multiple types of pediatric cancers. In general, carboplatin induces mild to moderate hypersensitivity reactions, although it is well recognized that anaphylaxis can occur. The incidence of severe carboplatin hypersensitivity in children has been reported to range from 4% to 8%.[86,87] Most reactions are early onset and thought to be IgE mediated.[81,88] However, delayed onset reactions occurring hours to days later have rarely been reported.[80,81] As in adults, carboplatin-induced hypersensitivity typically manifests after multiple cycles, with most pediatric reactions occurring during the eighth cycle.[89,90] Repeated exposure increases the risk of reaction. Genc and colleagues[89] identified weekly carboplatin infusions, younger age, and female gender as risk factors for reactions in pediatric patients with brain tumors. Management options include drug discontinuation, substitution with another platinum-based drug, and desensitization. Switching from carboplatin to cisplatin may not be feasible owing to cross-reactivity between the 2 compounds, although the incidence of carboplatin and cisplatin cross-reactivity has not been well defined.[80] Oxaliplatin reaction rates are lower but may be rising with increased use of the drug.[81]

Skin testing has been shown to be useful for carboplatin-induced hypersensitivity, and the recommended concentration for epicutaneous testing is 10 mg/mL and up to 5 mg/mL for intradermal testing.[91] Multiple cases of successful carboplatin desensitizations have been reported in pediatric patients.[92–94] Rodriguez Del Rio and colleagues[94] used a slightly modified version of the 12-step protocol published by Castells and colleagues[84] to desensitize 7 patients with low-grade gliomas.[84] In addition, a modified carboplatin desensitization protocol has been described by Lazzareschi and colleagues,[86] in which 6 children were successfully desensitized without use of premedications.[86] Sims-McCallum and colleagues[92] also reported the case of a 10-year-old female patient with bilateral optic glioma who underwent successful inpatient carboplatin desensitization and was subsequently able to receive carboplatin desensitization and treatment in the outpatient infusion center, with appropriate monitoring.

L-ASPARAGINASE (NATIVE *ESCHERICHIA COLI* ASPARAGINASE, PEGYLATED-ASPARAGINASE, *ERWINIA* ASPARAGINASE)

L-Asparaginase is particularly important in the treatment of acute lymphoblastic leukemia, and hypersensitivity reactions are relatively common. The 3 preparations commercially available in the United States are derived from bacterial sources. Hypersensitivity reactions to pegylated (PEG)-asparaginase are least frequent and range from 3% to 24%. Risk of hypersensitivity to PEG-asparaginase increases with prior exposure to native *Escherichia coli* asparaginase, because of their shared bacterial source.[95] Most reactions are immediate and are thought to be either IgE induced or related to IgM- or IgG-induced complement activation.[81,88] Hypersensitivity reactions have been reported after the first dose but are more common with repeated doses, especially with reintroduction or dosing intervals of a week or longer.[79,88] Administration is almost never via the intravenous route owing to higher rates of hypersensitivity.

Patients who display hypersensitivity to L-asparaginase should generally be switched to an alternate preparation; those with native L-asparaginase hypersensitivity can often tolerate PEG-asparaginase, and those with *E coli*–derived asparaginase hypersensitivity can be switched to *Erwinia* asparaginase. It should be noted, however, that cross-reactivity between *E coli* and *Erwinia* derivatives has been reported.[96]

Skin testing is not standardized and is of limited value because it may produce false negatives. The recommended amount is 0.1 mL intradermally of a 20-IU dilution of the drug. Test doses are of limited value because small doses rarely produce a reaction.[88] Desensitization is also an option and has been successfully performed.[80,81,97]

METHOTREXATE

Methotrexate is widely used in pediatric blood cancers and osteosarcoma. Hypersensitivity reactions are rare, and severe reactions are reported in less than 1% of cases.[80] Most reactions are thought to be IgE mediated, although anaphylactoid reactions have been reported.[98] Reactions can range from mild to life threatening. Skin tests have not routinely been performed owing to the high frequency of negative results,[80,85] and the few case reports detailing methotrexate desensitizations have used prolonged infusions.[80,81,98,99] However, Dilley and colleagues[100] recently published a novel case series describing skin testing, graded challenge, and desensitization to methotrexate in 7 pediatric patients. Four patients who did not require urgent drug administration underwent skin prick testing to methotrexate, which was performed at a concentration of 10 mg/mL followed by intradermal testing with 0.1-mg/mL, 1-mg/mL, and 10-mg/mL concentrations. One patient with a history of mild reaction and negative skin test tolerated graded challenge. A total of 17 desensitizations were performed in the remaining 6 patients. Most patients successfully underwent 12-step desensitization protocol; 1 patient who did not was able to tolerate a 16-step protocol.

ANTHRACYCLINES (DAUNORUBICIN, DOXORUBICIN, AND EPIRUBICIN)

Anthracyclines are used with multiple types of pediatric cancers, but hypersensitivity reactions are rare. Skin testing is not typically performed due to cutaneous toxicity.[85] Premedication is often not useful, but slowing the infusion rate, especially with the PEG liposomal formulation, which can induce rapid-onset symptoms, can produce good results.[80]

VINCA ALKALOIDS (VINCRISTINE, VINBLASTINE)

Vincristine is used widely in pediatric cancers, but hypersensitivity reactions are very rarely reported. Interestingly, Hill and colleagues[101] recently reported 8 patients with reactions to vincristine, consistent with anecdotal reactions at other institutions. Mass spectrometry of medication lots was concerning for possible contaminant. Skin testing to vincristine is not performed due to irritant reactions. Case reports of desensitization have been published.[93]

SUMMARY

BL antibiotics and NSAIDs remain the most common causes of pediatric drug hypersensitivity, although only a minority of reactions is generally confirmed as true drug allergy. Evaluation of penicillin allergy in children, especially those considered low risk, is trending away from skin testing and toward direct drug provocation challenge, although it is unclear whether this is also the best method for adolescents. The utility of prolonged challenges has also been addressed. Regarding NSAID hypersensitivity, the need for a pediatric-specific classification of NSAID hypersensitivity reactions has been recognized. Diagnosis typically requires drug challenges because of the lack of standardized and widely available in vivo and in vitro testing. Non-BL antibiotics are less common but still noteworthy causes of pediatric hypersensitivity reactions. Nonirritating skin test concentrations have been published but for the most part have not yet been validated in children. In the realm of chemotherapeutics, hypersensitivity to platinum-based drugs and L-asparaginase occurs relatively frequently; skin testing to carboplatin has been shown to be useful, and desensitization is a feasible option. Overall, an understanding of pediatric drug allergies and confirmation through accepted diagnostic methods is crucial to prevent overdiagnosis.

REFERENCES

1. Smyth RM, Gargon E, Kirkham J, et al. Adverse drug reactions in children—a systematic review. PLoS One 2012;7(3):e24061.
2. Erkocoglu M, Kaya A, Civelek E, et al. Prevalence of confirmed immediate type drug hypersensitivity reactions among school children. Pediatr Allergy Immunol 2013;24(2):160–7.
3. Gomes ER, Brockow K, Kuyucu S, et al. Drug hypersensitivity in children: report from the pediatric task force of the EAACI Drug Allergy Interest Group. Allergy 2016;71(2):149–61.
4. Langley JM, Halperin SA, Bortolussi R. History of penicillin allergy and referral for skin testing: evaluation of a pediatric penicillin allergy testing program. Clin Invest Med 2002;25(5):181–4.
5. Lucas M, Arnold A, Sommerfield A, et al. Antibiotic allergy labels in children are associated with adverse clinical outcomes. J Allergy Clin Immunol Pract 2018. https://doi.org/10.1016/j.jaip.2018.09.003.
6. Ponvert C, Perrin Y, Bados-Albiero A, et al. Allergy to betalactam antibiotics in children: results of a 20-year study based on clinical history, skin and challenge tests. Pediatr Allergy Immunol 2011;22(4):411–8.
7. Ponvert C, Weilenmann C, Wassenberg J, et al. Allergy to betalactam antibiotics in children: a prospective follow-up study in retreated children after negative responses in skin and challenge tests. Allergy 2007;62(1):42–6.
8. Allergic reactions to long-term benzathine penicillin prophylaxis for rheumatic fever. International Rheumatic Fever Study Group. Lancet 1991;337(8753): 1308–10.
9. Drug allergy: an updated practice parameter. Ann Allergy Asthma Immunol 2010;105(4):259–73.
10. Caubet JC, Kaiser L, Lemaitre B, et al. The role of penicillin in benign skin rashes in childhood: a prospective study based on drug rechallenge. J Allergy Clin Immunol 2011;127(1):218–22.
11. Dibek Misirlioglu E, Guvenir H, Ozkaya Parlakay A, et al. Incidence of antibiotic-related rash in children with Epstein-Barr virus infection and evaluation of the frequency of confirmed antibiotic hypersensitivity. Int Arch Allergy Immunol 2018; 176(1):33–8.
12. Demoly P, Adkinson NF, Brockow K, et al. International consensus on drug allergy. Allergy 2014;69(4):420–37.
13. Peter JG, Lehloenya R, Dlamini S, et al. Severe delayed cutaneous and systemic reactions to drugs: a global perspective on the science and art of current practice. J Allergy Clin Immunol Pract 2017;5(3):547–63.

14. Blanca M, Torres MJ, Garcia JJ, et al. Natural evolution of skin test sensitivity in patients allergic to beta-lactam antibiotics. J Allergy Clin Immunol 1999; 103(5 Pt 1):918–24.
15. Mill C, Primeau MN, Medoff E, et al. Assessing the diagnostic properties of a graded oral provocation challenge for the diagnosis of immediate and nonimmediate reactions to amoxicillin in children. JAMA Pediatr 2016;170(6): e160033.
16. Ibanez MD, Rodriguez Del Rio P, Lasa EM, et al. Prospective assessment of diagnostic tests for pediatric penicillin allergy: from clinical history to challenge tests. Ann Allergy Asthma Immunol 2018;121(2):235–44.e3.
17. Atanaskovic-Markovic M, Gaeta F, Medjo B, et al. Non-immediate hypersensitivity reactions to beta-lactam antibiotics in children—our 10-year experience in allergy work-up. Pediatr Allergy Immunol 2016;27(5):533–8.
18. Zambonino MA, Corzo JL, Munoz C, et al. Diagnostic evaluation of hypersensitivity reactions to beta-lactam antibiotics in a large population of children. Pediatr Allergy Immunol 2014;25(1):80–7.
19. Confino-Cohen R, Rosman Y, Meir-Shafrir K, et al. Oral challenge without skin testing safely excludes clinically significant delayed-onset penicillin hypersensitivity. J Allergy Clin Immunol Pract 2017;5(3):669–75.
20. Mori F, Cianferoni A, Barni S, et al. Amoxicillin allergy in children: five-day drug provocation test in the diagnosis of nonimmediate reactions. J Allergy Clin Immunol Pract 2015;3(3):375–80.e1.
21. Vezir E, Dibek Misirlioglu E, Civelek E, et al. Direct oral provocation tests in nonimmediate mild cutaneous reactions related to beta-lactam antibiotics. Pediatr Allergy Immunol 2016;27(1):50–4.
22. Iammatteo M, Alvarez Arango S, Ferastraoaru D, et al. Safety and outcomes of oral graded challenges to amoxicillin without prior skin testing. J Allergy Clin Immunol Pract 2018. https://doi.org/10.1016/j.jaip.2018.05.008.
23. Labrosse R, Paradis L, Lacombe-Barrios J, et al. Efficacy and safety of 5-day challenge for the evaluation of nonsevere amoxicillin allergy in children. J Allergy Clin Immunol Pract 2018;6(5):1673–80.
24. Blanca-Lopez N, Zapatero L, Alonso E, et al. Skin testing and drug provocation in the diagnosis of nonimmediate reactions to aminopenicillins in children. Allergy 2009;64(2):229–33.
25. Garcia Rodriguez R, Moreno Lozano L, Extremera Ortega A, et al. Provocation tests in nonimmediate hypersensitivity reactions to beta-lactam antibiotics in children: are extended challenges needed? J Allergy Clin Immunol Pract 2018. https://doi.org/10.1016/j.jaip.2018.06.023.
26. Picard M, Paradis L, Nguyen M, et al. Outpatient penicillin use after negative skin testing and drug challenge in a pediatric population. Allergy Asthma Proc 2012;33(2):160–4.
27. Roehmel JF, Schwarz C, Mehl A, et al. Hypersensitivity to antibiotics in patients with cystic fibrosis. J Cyst Fibros 2014;13(2):205–11.
28. Matar R, Le Bourgeois M, Scheinmann P, et al. Beta-lactam hypersensitivity in children with cystic fibrosis: a study in a specialized pediatric center for cystic fibrosis and drug allergy. Pediatr Allergy Immunol 2014;25(1):88–93.
29. Sullivan TJ, Yecies LD, Shatz GS, et al. Desensitization of patients allergic to penicillin using orally administered beta-lactam antibiotics. J Allergy Clin Immunol 1982;69(3):275–82.
30. Cernadas JR. Desensitization to antibiotics in children. Pediatr Allergy Immunol 2013;24(1):3–9.

31. Solensky R. Drug desensitization. Immunol Allergy Clin North Am 2004;24(3): 425–43, vi.

32. De Maria C, Lebel D, Desroches A, et al. Simple intravenous antimicrobial desensitization method for pediatric patients. Am J Health Syst Pharm 2002; 59(16):1532–6.

33. Kidon M, Blanca-Lopez N, Gomes E, et al. EAACI/ENDA position paper: diagnosis and management of hypersensitivity reactions to non-steroidal anti-inflammatory drugs (NSAIDs) in children and adolescents. Pediatr Allergy Immunol 2018;29(5):469–80.

34. Rubio M, Bousquet PJ, Gomes E, et al. Results of drug hypersensitivity evaluations in a large group of children and adults. Clin Exp Allergy 2012;42(1):123–30.

35. Cousin M, Chiriac A, Molinari N, et al. Phenotypical characterization of children with hypersensitivity reactions to NSAIDs. Pediatr Allergy Immunol 2016;27(7): 743–8.

36. Blanca-Lopez N, Pérez-Alzate D, Cornejo JA, et al. Hypersensitivity reactions to NSAIDs in children. J Allergy Clin Immunol 2017;139(2):AB34.

37. Corzo JL, Zambonino MA, Munoz C, et al. Tolerance to COX-2 inhibitors in children with hypersensitivity to nonsteroidal anti-inflammatory drugs. Br J Dermatol 2014;170(3):725–9.

38. Zambonino MA, Torres MJ, Munoz C, et al. Drug provocation tests in the diagnosis of hypersensitivity reactions to non-steroidal anti-inflammatory drugs in children. Pediatr Allergy Immunol 2013;24(2):151–9.

39. Kowalski ML, Asero R, Bavbek S, et al. Classification and practical approach to the diagnosis and management of hypersensitivity to nonsteroidal anti-inflammatory drugs. Allergy 2013;68(10):1219–32.

40. Himly M, Jahn-Schmid B, Pittertschatscher K, et al. IgE-mediated immediate-type hypersensitivity to the pyrazolone drug propyphenazone. J Allergy Clin Immunol 2003;111(4):882–8.

41. Cavkaytar O, Arik Yilmaz E, Karaatmaca B, et al. Different phenotypes of nonsteroidal anti-inflammatory drug hypersensitivity during childhood. Int Arch Allergy Immunol 2015;167(3):211–21.

42. Yilmaz O, Ertoy Karagol IH, Bakirtas A, et al. Challenge-proven nonsteroidal anti-inflammatory drug hypersensitivity in children. Allergy 2013;68(12): 1555–61.

43. Mayorga C, Sanz ML, Gamboa P, et al. In vitro methods for diagnosing nonimmediate hypersensitivity reactions to drugs. J Investig Allergol Clin Immunol 2013;23(4):213–25 [quiz precedeing 25].

44. Cavkaytar O, Arik Yilmaz E, Buyuktiryaki B, et al. Challenge-proven aspirin hypersensitivity in children with chronic spontaneous urticaria. Allergy 2015; 70(2):153–60.

45. Lee RU, Stevenson DD. Aspirin-exacerbated respiratory disease: evaluation and management. Allergy Asthma Immunol Res 2011;3(1):3–10.

46. Lo PC, Tsai YT, Lin SK, et al. Risk of asthma exacerbation associated with nonsteroidal anti-inflammatory drugs in childhood asthma: a nationwide population-based cohort study in Taiwan. Medicine 2016;95(41):e5109.

47. Debley JS, Carter ER, Gibson RL, et al. The prevalence of ibuprofen-sensitive asthma in children: a randomized controlled bronchoprovocation challenge study. J Pediatr 2005;147(2):233–8.

48. Asaumi T, Yanagida N, Sato S, et al. Provocation tests for the diagnosis of food-dependent exercise-induced anaphylaxis. Pediatr Allergy Immunol 2016;27(1):44–9.

49. Ameratunga R, Randall N, Dalziel S, et al. Samter's triad in childhood: a warning for those prescribing NSAIDs. Paediatr Anaesth 2013;23(8):757–9.

50. Ertoy Karagol HI, Yilmaz O, Topal E, et al. Nonsteroidal anti-inflammatory drugs-exacerbated respiratory disease in adolescents. Int Forum Allergy Rhinol 2015; 5(5):392–8.

51. Tuttle KL, Schneider TR, Henrickson SE, et al. Aspirin-exacerbated respiratory disease: not always "adult-onset". J Allergy Clin Immunol Pract 2016;4(4):756–8.

52. Lee RU, White AA, Ding D, et al. Use of intranasal ketorolac and modified oral aspirin challenge for desensitization of aspirin-exacerbated respiratory disease. Ann Allergy Asthma Immunol 2010;105(2):130–5.

53. Empedrad R, Darter AL, Earl HS, et al. Nonirritating intradermal skin test concentrations for commonly prescribed antibiotics. J Allergy Clin Immunol 2003; 112(3):629–30.

54. Sanchez-Borges M, Thong B, Blanca M, et al. Hypersensitivity reactions to non beta-lactam antimicrobial agents, a statement of the WAO special committee on drug allergy. World Allergy Organ J 2013;6(1):18.

55. Kuyucu S, Mori F, Atanaskovic-Markovic M, et al. Hypersensitivity reactions to non-betalactam antibiotics in children: an extensive review. Pediatr Allergy Immunol 2014;25(6):534–43.

56. Guvenir H, Dibek Misirlioglu E, Capanoglu M, et al. Proven non-beta-lactam antibiotic allergy in children. Int Arch Allergy Immunol 2016;169(1):45–50.

57. Levi N, Bastuji-Garin S, Mockenhaupt M, et al. Medications as risk factors of Stevens-Johnson syndrome and toxic epidermal necrolysis in children: a pooled analysis. Pediatrics 2009;123(2):e297–304.

58. Kreuz W, Gungor T, Lotz C, et al. "Treating through" hypersensitivity to cotrimoxazole in children with HIV infection. Lancet 1990;336(8713):508–9.

59. Gomez-Traseira C, Boyano-Martinez T, Escosa-Garcia L, et al. Trimethoprim-sulfamethoxazole (cotrimoxazole) desensitization in an HIV-infected 5-yr-old girl. Pediatr Allergy Immunol 2015;26(3):287–9.

60. D'Amelio CM, Del Pozo JL, Vega O, et al. Successful desensitization in a child with delayed cotrimoxazole hypersensitivity: a case report. Pediatr Allergy Immunol 2016;27(3):320–1.

61. Straatmann A, Bahia F, Pedral-Sampaio D, et al. A randomized, pilot trial comparing full versus escalating dose regimens for the desensitization of AIDS patients allergic to sulfonamides. Braz J Infect Dis 2002;6(6):276–80.

62. Bonfanti P, Pusterla L, Parazzini F, et al. The effectiveness of desensitization versus rechallenge treatment in HIV-positive patients with previous hypersensitivity to TMP-SMX: a randomized multicentric study. C.I.S.A.I. Group. Biomed Pharmacother 2000;54(1):45–9.

63. Leoung GS, Stanford JF, Giordano MF, et al. Trimethoprim-sulfamethoxazole (TMP-SMZ) dose escalation versus direct rechallenge for Pneumocystis Carinii pneumonia prophylaxis in human immunodeficiency virus-infected patients with previous adverse reaction to TMP-SMZ. J Infect Dis 2001;184(8):992–7.

64. Benahmed S, Scaramuzza C, Messaad D, et al. The accuracy of the diagnosis of suspected macrolide antibiotic hypersensitivity: results of a single-blinded trial. Allergy 2004;59(10):1130–3.

65. Mori F, Barni S, Pucci N, et al. Sensitivity and specificity of skin tests in the diagnosis of clarithromycin allergy. Ann Allergy Asthma Immunol 2010;104(5):417–9.

66. Macy E, Romano A, Khan D. Practical management of antibiotic hypersensitivity in 2017. J Allergy Clin Immunol Pract 2017;5(3):577–86.

67. Mori F, Pecorari L, Pantano S, et al. Azithromycin anaphylaxis in children. Int J Immunopathol Pharmacol 2014;27(1):121–6.
68. Swamy N, Laurie SA, Ruiz-Huidobro E, et al. Successful clarithromycin desensitization in a multiple macrolide-allergic patient. Ann Allergy Asthma Immunol 2010;105(6):489–90.
69. Petitto J, Chervinskiy SK, Scurlock AM, et al. Successful clarithromycin desensitization in a macrolide-sensitive pediatric patient. J Allergy Clin Immunol Pract 2013;1(3):307–8.
70. Kendigelen P, BaktirClinic Of Anesthesiology And Reanimation Afşin State Hospital Afşin Kahramanmaraş Tureky M, Sucu A, et al. Anaphylaxis after administration of amikacin containing sodium metabisulfite in a premature newborn. Arch Argent Pediatr 2016;114(3):e195–8.
71. Belloni Fortina A, Romano I, Peserico A, et al. Contact sensitization in very young children. J Am Acad Dermatol 2011;65(4):772–9.
72. Spigarelli MG, Hurwitz ME, Nasr SZ. Hypersensitivity to inhaled TOBI following reaction to gentamicin. Pediatr Pulmonol 2002;33(4):311–4.
73. Earl HS, Sullivan TJ. Acute desensitization of a patient with cystic fibrosis allergic to both beta-lactam and aminoglycoside antibiotics. J Allergy Clin Immunol 1987;79(3):477–83.
74. Schretlen-Doherty JS, Troutman WG. Tobramycin-induced hypersensitivity reaction. Ann Pharmacother 1995;29(7–8):704–6.
75. Etminan M, Guo M, Carleton B. Oral fluoroquinolone prescribing to children in the United States from 2006 to 2015. Pediatr Infect Dis J 2018. https://doi.org/10.1097/inf.0000000000002121.
76. Lantner RR. Ciprofloxacin desensitization in a patient with cystic fibrosis. J Allergy Clin Immunol 1995;96(6 Pt 1):1001–2.
77. Erdem G, Staat MA, Connelly BL, et al. Anaphylactic reaction to ciprofloxacin in a toddler: successful desensitization. Pediatr Infect Dis J 1999;18(6):563–4.
78. Dubini M, Marraccini P, Pignatti P. Multiple drug allergy: a case of anaphylaxis to levofloxacin but tolerance to ciprofloxacin. Ann Allergy Asthma Immunol 2016;116(5):465.
79. Young JS, Simmons JW. Chemotherapeutic medications and their emergent complications. Hematol Oncol Clin North Am 2017;31(6):995–1010.
80. Ruggiero A, Triarico S, Trombatore G, et al. Incidence, clinical features and management of hypersensitivity reactions to chemotherapeutic drugs in children with cancer. Eur J Clin Pharmacol 2013;69(10):1739–46.
81. Cernadas JR. Reactions to cytostatic agents in children. Curr Opin Allergy Clin Immunol 2017;17(4):255–61.
82. Webber KA, Kos L, Holland KE, et al. Intertriginous eruption associated with chemotherapy in pediatric patients. Arch Dermatol 2007;143(1):67–71.
83. Lim D, Aussedat M, Maillet-Lebel N, et al. Flagellate dermatitis in a child most likely secondary to doxorubicin. Pediatr Dermatol 2017;34(5):e257–9.
84. Castells MC, Tennant NM, Sloane DE, et al. Hypersensitivity reactions to chemotherapy: outcomes and safety of rapid desensitization in 413 cases. J Allergy Clin Immunol 2008;122(3):574–80.
85. Hong DI, Dioun AF. Indications, protocols, and outcomes of drug desensitizations for chemotherapy and monoclonal antibodies in adults and children. J Allergy Clin Immunol Pract 2014;2(1):13–9 [quiz: 20].
86. Lazzareschi I, Ruggiero A, Riccardi R, et al. Hypersensitivity reactions to carboplatin in children. J Neurooncol 2002;58(1):33–7.

87. Lafay-Cousin L, Sung L, Carret AS, et al. Carboplatin hypersensitivity reaction in pediatric patients with low-grade glioma: a Canadian Pediatric Brain Tumor Consortium experience. Cancer 2008;112(4):892–9.
88. Lee C, Gianos M, Klaustermeyer WB. Diagnosis and management of hypersensitivity reactions related to common cancer chemotherapy agents. Ann Allergy Asthma Immunol 2009;102(3):179–87 [quiz: 87–9, 222].
89. Genc DB, Canpolat C, Berrak SG. Clinical features and management of carboplatin-related hypersensitivity reactions in pediatric low-grade glioma. Support Care Cancer 2012;20(2):385–93.
90. Yu DY, Dahl GV, Shames RS, et al. Weekly dosing of carboplatin increases risk of allergy in children. J Pediatr Hematol Oncol 2001;23(6):349–52.
91. Lax T, Long A, Banerji A. Skin testing in the evaluation and management of carboplatin-related hypersensitivity reactions. J Allergy Clin Immunol Pract 2015;3(6):856–62.
92. Sims-McCallum RP. Outpatient carboplatin desensitization in a pediatric patient with bilateral optic glioma. Ann Pharmacother 2000;34(4):477–8.
93. Visitsunthorn N, Utsawapreechawong W, Pacharn P, et al. Immediate type hypersensitivity to chemotherapeutic agents in pediatric patients. Asian Pac J Allergy Immunol 2009;27(4):191–7.
94. Rodriguez Del Rio P, Andion M, Ruano D, et al. Initial experience with carboplatin desensitization: a case series in a paediatric hospital. Pediatr Allergy Immunol 2018;29(1):111–5.
95. Hijiya N, van der Sluis IM. Asparaginase-associated toxicity in children with acute lymphoblastic leukemia. Leuk Lymphoma 2016;57(4):748–57.
96. Vrooman LM, Supko JG, Neuberg DS, et al. Erwinia asparaginase after allergy to E. coli asparaginase in children with acute lymphoblastic leukemia. Pediatr Blood Cancer 2010;54(2):199–205.
97. Soyer OU, Aytac S, Tuncer A, et al. Alternative algorithm for L-asparaginase allergy in children with acute lymphoblastic leukemia. J Allergy Clin Immunol 2009;123(4):895–9.
98. Oulego-Erroz I, Maneiro-Freire M, Bouzon-Alejandro M, et al. Anaphylactoid reaction to high-dose methotrexate and successful desensitization. Pediatr Blood Cancer 2010;55(3):557–9.
99. Kohli A, Ferencz TM, Calderon JG. Readministration of high-dose methotrexate in a patient with suspected immediate hypersensitivity and T-cell acute lymphoblastic lymphoma. Allergy Asthma Proc 2004;25(4):249–52.
100. Dilley MA, Lee JP, Broyles AD. Methotrexate hypersensitivity reactions in pediatrics: evaluation and management. Pediatr Blood Cancer 2017;64(5). https://doi.org/10.1002/pbc.26306.
101. Hill DA, Leahy AB, Sciasci J, et al. Medication contaminants as a potential cause of anaphylaxis to vincristine. Pediatr Blood Cancer 2018;65(1). https://doi.org/10.1002/pbc.26761.

UNITED STATES POSTAL SERVICE® Statement of Ownership, Management, and Circulation (All Periodicals Publications Except Requester Publications)

1. Publication Title	2. Publication Number	3. Filing Date
PEDIATRIC CLINICS OF NORTH AMERICA	424 – 66	9/18/2019

4. Issue Frequency	5. Number of Issues Published Annually	6. Annual Subscription Price
FEB, APR, JUN, AUG, OCT, DEC	6	$229.00

7. Complete Mailing Address of Known Office of Publication (Not printer) (Street, city, county, state, and ZIP+4®)

ELSEVIER INC.
230 Park Avenue, Suite 800
New York, NY 10169

Contact Person
STEPHEN R. BUSHING

Telephone (Include area code)
215-239-3688

8. Complete Mailing Address of Headquarters or General Business Office of Publisher (Not printer)

ELSEVIER INC.
230 Park Avenue, Suite 800
New York, NY 10169

9. Full Names and Complete Mailing Addresses of Publisher, Editor, and Managing Editor (Do not leave blank)

Publisher (Name and complete mailing address)

TAYLOR BALL, ELSEVIER INC.
1600 JOHN F KENNEDY BLVD. SUITE 1800
PHILADELPHIA, PA 19103-2899

Editor (Name and complete mailing address)

KERRY HOLLAND, ELSEVIER INC.
1600 JOHN F KENNEDY BLVD. SUITE 1800
PHILADELPHIA, PA 19103-2899

Managing Editor (Name and complete mailing address)

PATRICK MANLEY, ELSEVIER INC.
1600 JOHN F KENNEDY BLVD. SUITE 1800
PHILADELPHIA, PA 19103-2899

10. Owner (Do not leave blank. If the publication is owned by a corporation, give the name and address of the corporation immediately followed by the names and addresses of all stockholders owning or holding 1 percent or more of the total amount of stock. If not owned by a corporation, give the names and addresses of the individual owners. If owned by a partnership or other unincorporated firm, give its name and address as well as those of each individual owner. If the publication is published by a nonprofit organization, give its name and address.)

Full Name	Complete Mailing Address
WHOLLY OWNED SUBSIDIARY OF REED/ELSEVIER, US HOLDINGS	1600 JOHN F KENNEDY BLVD. SUITE 1800 PHILADELPHIA, PA 19103-2899

11. Known Bondholders, Mortgagees, and Other Security Holders Owning or Holding 1 Percent or More of Total Amount of Bonds, Mortgages, or Other Securities. If none, check box ▶ ☐ None

Full Name	Complete Mailing Address
N/A	

12. Tax Status (For completion by nonprofit organizations authorized to mail at nonprofit rates) (Check one)
The purpose, function, and nonprofit status of this organization and the exempt status for federal income tax purposes:
☒ Has Not Changed During Preceding 12 Months
☐ Has Changed During Preceding 12 Months (Publisher must submit explanation of change with this statement)

PS Form 3526, July 2014 [Page 1 of 4 (see instructions page 4)] PSN: 7530-01-000-9931 PRIVACY NOTICE: See our privacy policy on www.usps.com.

13. Publication Title		14. Issue Date for Circulation Data Below
PEDIATRIC CLINICS OF NORTH AMERICA		AUGUST 2019

15. Extent and Nature of Circulation			Average No. Copies Each Issue During Preceding 12 Months	No. Copies of Single Issue Published Nearest to Filing Date
a. Total Number of Copies (Net press run)			535	651
b. Paid Circulation (By Mail and Outside the Mail)	(1)	Mailed Outside-County Paid Subscriptions Stated on PS Form 3541 (Include paid distribution above nominal rate, advertiser's proof copies, and exchange copies)	246	168
	(2)	Mailed In-County Paid Subscriptions Stated on PS Form 3541 (Include paid distribution above nominal rate, advertiser's proof copies, and exchange copies)	0	0
	(3)	Paid Distribution Outside the Mails Including Sales Through Dealers and Carriers, Street Vendors, Counter Sales, and Other Paid Distribution Outside USPS®	197	249
	(4)	Paid Distribution by Other Classes of Mail Through the USPS (e.g., First-Class Mail®)	0	0
c. Total Paid Distribution (Sum of 15b (1), (2), (3), and (4))			443	417
d. Free or Nominal Rate Distribution (By Mail and Outside the Mail)	(1)	Free or Nominal Rate Outside-County Copies Included on PS Form 3541	78	217
	(2)	Free or Nominal Rate In-County Copies Included on PS Form 3541	0	0
	(3)	Free or Nominal Rate Copies Mailed at Other Classes Through the USPS (e.g., First-Class Mail)	0	0
	(4)	Free or Nominal Rate Distribution Outside the Mail (Carriers or other means)	0	0
e. Total Free or Nominal Rate Distribution (Sum of 15d (1), (2), (3) and (4))			78	217
f. Total Distribution (Sum of 15c and 15e)			521	634
g. Copies not Distributed (See Instructions to Publishers #4 (page #3))			14	17
h. Total (Sum of 15f and g)			535	651
i. Percent Paid (15c divided by 15f times 100)			85.03%	65.77%

* If you are claiming electronic copies, go to line 16 on page 3. If you are not claiming electronic copies, skip to line 17 on page 3.

16. Electronic Copy Circulation	Average No. Copies Each Issue During Preceding 12 Months	No. Copies of Single Issue Published Nearest to Filing Date
a. Paid Electronic Copies	▲	
b. Total Print Copies (Line 15c) + Paid Electronic Copies (Line 16a)	▲	
c. Total Print Distribution (Line 15f) + Paid Electronic Copies (Line 16a)	▲	
d. Percent Paid (Both Print & Electronic Copies) (16b divided by 16c × 100)	▲	

☒ I certify that 50% of all my distributed copies (electronic and print) are paid above a nominal price.

17. Publication of Statement of Ownership
☒ If the publication is a general publication, publication of this statement is required. Will be printed ☐ Publication not required.
in the OCTOBER 2019 issue of this publication.

18. Signature and Title of Editor, Publisher, Business Manager, or Owner

STEPHEN R. BUSHING, INVENTORY DISTRIBUTION CONTROL MANAGER

Stephen R. Bushing Date 9/18/2019

I certify that all information furnished on this form is true and complete. I understand that anyone who furnishes false or misleading information on this form or who omits material or information requested on the form may be subject to criminal sanctions (including fines and imprisonment) and/or civil sanctions (including civil penalties).

PS Form 3526, July 2014 (Page 3 of 4) PRIVACY NOTICE: See our privacy policy on www.usps.com.

Moving?

Make sure your subscription moves with you!

To notify us of your new address, find your **Clinics Account Number** (located on your mailing label above your name), and contact customer service at:

Email: journalscustomerservice-usa@elsevier.com

800-654-2452 (subscribers in the U.S. & Canada)
314-447-8871 (subscribers outside of the U.S. & Canada)

Fax number: 314-447-8029

Elsevier Health Sciences Division
Subscription Customer Service
3251 Riverport Lane
Maryland Heights, MO 63043

*To ensure uninterrupted delivery of your subscription,
please notify us at least 4 weeks in advance of move.

Printed and bound by CPI Group (UK) Ltd, Croydon, CR0 4YY

03/10/2024

01040407-0014